An Electrophysiological Approach to the Diagnosis of Arrhythmias

1: Tachycardia

Christopher R.C. Wyndham, M.D.
Director of Cardiac Electrophysiology
Director of Electrocardiology
Presbyterian Hospital of Dallas
and
Clinical Professor of Medicine
Southwestern Medical School
University of Texas Health Sciences Center
Dallas, Texas

FUTURA

**Futura Publishing
Company, Inc.**
Mount Kisco, NY
1991

Copyright © 1991
Published by
Futura Publishing Company, Inc.
2 Bedford Ridge Road
Mount Kisco, New York 10549
ISBN: 0-87993-501-4
ISSN: 1053-8437

Acknowledgments

The author records his indebtedness to the support, stimulus, and continuing encouragement of Sharon Magro, P.A.C and of the many Fellows in Electrophysiology at the University of Illinois, Baylor College of Medicine, and at Southwestern Medical School. The manuscript was expertly prepared by Kalene Farley and Phyllis Jarrett, whose care and dedication are unequaled. The photographs were prepared by Rick Smith, Supervisor of Media Services at Presbyterian Hospital of Dallas.

Contents

Introduction

Electrophysiological studies have taught us much about the mechanisms of paroxysmal tachycardias. While there is still much to be discovered, especially the detailed microscopic and cellular basis of arrhythmias, many practical rules have been derived and validated. These rules are helpful in elucidating the mechanism of paroxysmal tachycardias. An understanding of tachycardia mechanism—and how programmed electrical stimulation of the heart can prove the mechanism—can lead to a planned approach to rational therapy, be it emergency therapy or long term, and whether it be by pharmacologic means, by ablative or surgical means, or by the use of antitachycardia pacemakers or implantable antitachycardia devices with a broad range of programmable functions.

While successful therapy is the ultimate goal, accurate diagnosis should always be sought first, with the techniques immediately available to the emergency physician or with the more sophisticated techniques used more electively by the electrophysiologist.

This small text is not meant to be a primer in clinical cardiac electrophysiology. It is, rather, a somewhat organized, programmed text by which a stepwise approach can be made to the diagnosis of a paroxysmal tachycardia. Not all of the diagnostic steps can necessarily be taken during the acute presentation of a patient severely compromised by tachycardia. However one should proceed in a logical sequence. The utility of a full 12-lead electrocardiogram (ECG) cannot be overemphasized. It contains enormous information on atrioventricular relationships, P wave vector, and QRS morphology, that together contribute perhaps the most important information in seeking a diagnosis. A coordinated attempt at diagnosis should always precede therapy, if only to prevent drugs being given that may endanger the life or well being of the patient. An example is the rather frequent injudicious use of verapamil in patients with wide QRS tachycardia. A wide QRS tachycardia should always be assumed to be ventricular tachycardia unless unequivocally proved otherwise. A patient may walk into an emergency room in ventricular tachycardia and be in shock after the administration of a negative inotropic antiarrhythmic drug only minutes later unless a concerted effort is made to establish the diagnosis before treatment is initiated.

The diagnostic approach suggested here involves the use of clinical history, physical examination, analysis of the 12-lead ECG, esophageal or atrial electrograms, His bundle recordings, atrial and ventricular programmed stimulation, bedside maneuvers, and judicious administration of antiarrhythmic drugs. Not all of these maneuvers may be necessary or available in every case. However, the physician should be guided to appropriate use of invasive diagnostic techniques when indicated.

A. Use of the History in Diagnosis of Paroxysmal Tachycardia

While all varieties of paroxysmal tachyarrhythmias can occur in all clinical settings, there are some clinical rules that are helpful.

- A wide QRS tachycardia in an adult patient with underlying heart disease, especially previous myocardial infarction, is usually ventricular tachycardia.

- A patient with no previous history of heart disease and no evidence of such on physical examination usually will be found to have paroxysmal reentrant supraventricular tachycardia or perhaps atrial flutter or atrial fibrillation.

- A patient with known Wolff-Parkinson-White (WPW) syndrome usually presents with paroxysmal reentrant supraventricular tachycardia or atrial fibrillation.

- The nature of drugs previously prescribed to a patient for tachycardias should not be used as evidence of tachycardia mechanism. Thus, the prior use of verapamil does not necessarily imply the presence of supraventricular tachycardia, nor does the use of quinidine suggest ventricular tachycardia.

- However, successful use of drugs in the past for the interruption or prevention of tachycardias should be noted, since this fact may be very useful in controlling the episode with which the patient currently presents.

- Careful note should also be made of adverse effects of previously administered antiarrhythmic or other drugs.

- Contrary to popular belief, the age of the patient has not been helpful in determining the diagnosis, aside from the fact that atrial fibrillation and ventricular tachycardia are very rare in the first few years of life. As to the mechanism of a supraventricular tachycardia, young age of onset is not a reliable clue to the presence of a congenital accessory pathway. AV nodal reentrant SVT is as common a mechanism in the young as in the adult.

- Previous electrocardiograms are of great value, in sinus rhythm or in tachycardia. In sinus rhythm, one should note P wave morphology and axis, P-R interval, presence of previous myocardial infarction, intraventricular conduction defect, bundle branch block and fascicular blocks, frontal and horizontal plane QRS vectors, presence of delta waves, the presence of atrial or ventricular premature beats, and especially the QRS morphology of such complexes. During previously recorded tachycardias, concordance with features of the presenting arrhythmia should be confirmed. If the previous tachycardia has features different from the presenting arrhythmia, a unifying diagnosis should be sought.

- In planning therapy, it is necessary to note the previous frequency and duration of arrhythmic symptoms, the presence of syncope or other serious symptoms during tachycardia, the presence of known precipitating or ameliorating conditions or maneuvers, and the specific effects on frequency and duration of tachycardias by medications.

B. Use of Physical Examination in Diagnosis of Paroxysmal Tachycardia

While the patient is being attached to the ECG monitor there is usually time to obtain the salient features of the history mentioned above and to inspect the neck veins, auscultate for blood pressure, and examine the precordium.

- Patients who walk into emergency rooms with a good blood pressure and tolerating their tachycardia should not be assumed to have supraventricular arrhythmias.
- Regular cannon waves in the jugular veins during tachycardia are frequently seen in supraventricular tachycardia.
- Irregular cannon waves (when the variation is not simply a function of respiratory fluctuations) imply AV dissociation and therefore strongly suggest ventricular tachycardia.
- Sometimes, in atrial flutter or atrial fibrillation, low amplitude rapid "f" waves can be appreciated in the jugular veins.
- The arterial pressure is generally constant from beat to beat in supraventricular tachycardia or regularly conducted atrial flutter (for example, 2:1 conduction).
- Blood pressure is, of course, variable whenever there is variability in ventricular cycle length, as in atrial fibrillation.
- Pulsus alternans can be observed in many perfectly regular tachycardias, especially at high rates. A 2:1 electromechanical response sometimes occurs and can be confirmed by echocardiography.
- When arterial pulse pressure varies irregularly during a regular tachycardia, AV dissociation may be presumed. In the presence of a wide QRS, such a

finding is strongly suggestive of ventricular tachycardia.

- Auscultation of the precordium gives similar diagnostic information in that variation in the intensity of the first heart sound implies AV dissociation if the tachycardia is regular.
- During paroxysmal SVT, the first heart sound may be loud and constant from beat to beat consistent with the hemodynamic basis of venous cannon waves.
- A uniformly soft first heart sound has no diagnostic value during tachycardia since this may reflect merely the decrease in stroke volume.
- The heart rate per se is useful only if 120 bpm or less. If so, ventricular tachycardia or accelerated junctional rhythm should be suspected (resolved by inspecting QRS duration). All rates above 120 bpm can be encountered with roughly equal frequency during supraventricular as in ventricular tachycardia.

C. Use of the Electrocardiogram and the Role of Electrophysiological Study in the Diagnosis of Paroxysmal Tachycardia

Table I should be followed carefully, paying particular attention to subtleties in the 12-lead ECG (e.g., retrograde P waves, subtle variations in QRS morphology), synthesizing data according to the various known mechanisms of tachycardia, and using suggested diagnostic maneuvers where indicated. After treating 1,000 patients along these lines, the process becomes second nature!

Table I. Diagnostic Approach to Paroxysmal Tachycardia

Question/Answer	Conclusion	Next Step
1. Is QRS wide?	→	12-lead ECG, Calipers
• ≦ 0.10 sec	Supraventricular tachycardia (except VT in children)	Go to 2,9
• 0.11 to 0.13 sec	Probably supraventricular tachycardia (except VT in children)	Go to 2,9
• ≧ 0.14 sec	Probably ventricular	Go to 2,10
2. Is tachycardia regular?	→	Calipers
• Precisely regular	Reentrant SVT, VT or atrial flutter	Go to 3
• Alternating long-short	Reentrant SVT or atrialflutter	Go to 3
• Group beating	Consider Wenckebach	Go to 3,4,5
• Chaotically irregular	Atrial fibrillation	Go to 3,5
3. Are P waves visible?	→	12-lead ECG
• Yes	→	Check P wave vector Go to 4

Table I. Diagnostic Approach to Paroxysmal Tachycardia—*(Continued)*

Question/Answer	Conclusion	Next Step
• No		Esophageal or atrial electrogram.
	→	Go to 5
4. P wave vector	→	12-lead ECG
• Normal	Sinus tachycardia *or* Sinoatrial reentrant SVT *or* Atrial automatic SVT	Go to 5
• About −90°	AV nodal reentrant SVT *or* Orthodromic SVT using posteroseptal accessorypathway *or* PJRT *or* Junctional tachycardia *or* VT with intact VA conduction	Go to 5
• About 120° to 210°	Orthodromic SVT using left free wall accessory pathway *or* Left atrial tachycardia	
• Anterior	Left atrial tachycardia	
• Posterior	Right atrial tachycardia	Go to 5
5. Timing of atrial activity		Measure R-P or V-A interval
(a) A-V ratio 1:1	→	
• P simultaneous with QRS	AV nodal reentrant SVT	Go to 6,9,11

Table I. Diagnostic Approach to Paroxysmal Tachycardia—*(Continued)*

Question/Answer	Conclusion	Next Step
• P precedes QRS ("long R-P")	Atrial automatic SVT *or* Atrial reentrant SVT *or* PJRT *or* AV nodal reentrant SVT of unusual variety	Go to 6,9,11
• P follows QRS ("short R-P")	Orthodromic reentrant SVT using accessory pathway *or* AV nodal reentrant SVT *or* VT with intact VA conduction	Go to 6,9,10,11
(b) A-V ratio > 1:1	(rules out participation of retrograde accessory pathway)	Measure atrial rate
• Atrial rate > 360	Atrial fibrillation	
• Atrial rate 240–360	Atrial flutter	
• Atrial rate < 240	Atrial tachycardia	Go to 6, Table II
(c) AV dissociation or AV ratio < 1:1		
• Narrow QRS	Junctional tachycardia	
• Wide QRS	Ventricular tachycardia	Go to 6
6. Onset of Tachycardia	→	Inspect P-QRS of first beat of tachycardia
(a) Timing of P-QRS at onset		

Table I. Diagnostic Approach to Paroxysmal Tachycardia—(Continued)

Question/Answer	Conclusion	Next Step
• P precedes narrow QRS		
Patient with WPW	Probably orthodromic SVT	Go to 5a,7,8,9
Patient without WPW	Atrial reentrant SVT *or* Atrial automatic SVT *or* AV nodal reentrant SVT *or* Orthodromic reentrant SVT	Go to 5a,7,8,9
• P precedes wide QRS		
Patient with WPW	Orthodromic SVT + BBB *or* Antidromic SVT *or* Atrial flutter or fibrillation	Go to 1,7
Patient without WPW	Orthodromic SVT + BBB *or* Atrial flutter or fibrillation + BBB *or* Ventricular tachycardia	Go to 1,7
• Wide QRS initiates tachycardia	VPB → reentrant SVT *or* VPB → VT	Go to 7
(b) Does tachycardia accelerate after onset?	→	Calipers
• Yes	Automatic tachycardia	
• No	Automatic or reentrant tachycardia	Go to 7

Table I. Diagnostic Approach to Paroxysmal Tachycardia—*(Continued)*

Question/Answer	Conclusion	Next Step
7. After onset, does QRS become or remain wide?		
• Yes	SVT + BBB *or* Antidromic SVT *or* Atrial flutter or fib + BBB *or* Preexcited atrial flutter or fib *or* Ventricular tachycardia	Go to 2,5,8
• No	SVT with narrow QRS	Go to 2,5,8
8. Spontaneous termination of tachycardia →		Inspect P-QRS of last beat of tachycardia
(a) Is P or atrial activity the *last* event? →		Careful inspection of ECG and/or atrial electrogram
• P the last event (rules out atrial tachycardia)	AV nodal reentrant SVT *or* Orthodromic SVT *or* Antidromic SVT *or* VT with intact VA conduction	Go to 5a,9
• QRS the last event	Atrial tachycardia *or* AV nodal reentrant SVT *or* Orthodromic SVT *or* Antidromic SVT *or* Ventricular tachycardia	Go to 5a,9
(b) Does tachycardia slow down before termination? →		Calipers

Table I. Diagnostic Approach to Paroxysmal Tachycardia—*(Continued)*

Question/Answer	Conclusion	Next Step
• Yes	Automatic atrial tachycardia *or* AV nodal reentrant SVT *or* Orthodromic reentrant SVT *or* Ventricular tachycardia	Go to 5,9,10
• No	Most tachycardias	Go to 5,9,10

9. Analysis of QRS complex during SVT (QRS < 0.14 sec)

(a) Does QRS in SVT exactly reproduce QRS during NSR?   →   12-lead ECG

• Yes (rules out VT)	All forms of SVT, atrial flutter or fibrillation	
• No. During SVT there is:		
— New R' in V_1	AV nodal reentrant SVT	Go to 5a,9d
— Subtle shift in terminal QRS vector	AV nodal reentrant SVT	Go to 5a,9d
— No longer delta waves	Orthodromic SVT	Continue 9a
— QRS alternans	Orthodromic SVT *or* AV nodal reentrant SVT	Go to 9b
— Classical LBBB	Orthodromic SVT *or* Other SVTs	Go to 9b
— Classical RBBB	Orthodromic SVT *or* Other SVTs	Go to 9b

Table I. Diagnostic Approach to Paroxysmal Tachycardia—*(Continued)*		
Question/Answer	*Conclusion*	*Next Step*
(b) Check VA interval during BBB or fascicular block during tachycardia		
• VA interval longer with BBB or fascicular block relative to narrow QRS tachycardia	Orthodromic SVT using accessory pathway ipsilateral to blocked bundle branch or fascicle	Go to 11
(c) In patients with WPW, do initial QRS forces during tachycardia have same vector as patient's delta waves during NSR? →		Compare 12-lead ECGs
• No	Orthodromic SVT *or* Preexcited SVT using different accessory pathway *or* Ventricular tachycardia	Go to 5a,9d,9e,10
• Yes	Preexcited atrial flutter *or* Preexcited atrial fibrillation *or* Antidromic SVT *or* Preexcited atrial tach *or* AV nodal reentrant SVT + "bystander" accessory pathway *or* Mahaim fiber tachycardias	Go to 5a,5b
(d) In tachycardias with QRS 0.10 to 0.12 sec, resembling RBBB, are the following features present: Same axis as in NSR, rsR in V_1, Rs in V_6, rapid initial QRS forces?		

Table I. Diagnostic Approach to Paroxysmal Tachycardia—*(Continued)*

Question/Answer	Conclusion	Next Step
• Yes	Probably SVT + RBBB	Go to 5a,11
• No (any 2)	Consider VT	Atrial electrogram Go to 5c,10

(e) In tachycardias with QRS 0.10 to 0.12 sec, resembling LBBB, are the following features present: Same axis as in NSR, rS or QS in V_1, R in V_6, absence of q in I, aVL, V_5,V_6?

• Yes	Probably SVT + LBBB	
• No (any 1)	Consider VT	Atrial electrogram Go to 5c,10

10. Analysis of wide QRS during tachycardia in patients without WPW

(a) Is QRS $\geqq$ 0.14

sec?	→	12-lead ECG
• No	→	Go to 9d,9e,11
• Yes	→	Go to 10b,10c

(b) During tachycardia with QRS mainly upright in V_1, are following features present: Slurred initial QRS forces; monophasic or diphasic QRS in all leads; QS, rS, R or qR in V_6; different axis from NSR (especially superior); precordial concordance?

• Yes	Almost certainly VT	Go to 11
• No (any 1)	Probably VT but consider preexicted tachycardia or SVT with gross IVCD	Go to 5a,5b,11

(c) During tachycardia with mainly negative QRS in V_1, are following features present: broad initial r, RS, Qr in V_1; precordial concordance; qR, Q, Rs, RS in V_6; different axis from NSR?

• Yes	Almost certainly VT	Go to 11
• No (any 1)	Probably VT but	

Table I. Diagnostic Approach to Paroxysmal Tachycardia—(Continued)

Question/Answer	Conclusion	Next Step
	consider preexcited tachycardia *or* SVT with gross IVCD	Go to 5a,5b,11

11. If, after analysis of 12-lead ECG, atrial electrograms and initiation and termination of tachycardia, mechanism is still equivocal, then His bundle recording, mapping of atrial activation sequence and programmed atrial and ventricular stimulation will be necessary for complete diagnosis.

(a) His bundle potential precedes each QRS during tachycardia?

• Yes: HV ≧ HV in MSR:	Supraventricular tachycardia *or* BB reentrant VT	
HV < HV in NSR	VT with retrograde HPS conduction *or*	Go to 11b
	Atrial tach with maximal preexcitation	Go to 11b
• No: HV dissociation	Ventricular tachycardia	Go to 21

(b) Atrial activation begins in mid, lateral coronary sinus

• Yes	SVT (*or* VT) conducting via left free wall accessory pathway *or* Left atrial tachycardia	Go to 12

(c) Atrial activation begins in proximal or ostial coronary sinus

• Yes	SVT (*or* VT) conducting via left paraseptal *or* posterior septal accessory pathway *or*

Table I. Diagnostic Approach to Paroxysmal Tachycardia—*(Continued)*

Question/Answer	Conclusion	Next Step
	AV nodal reentrant SVT *or* Atrial septal tachycardia	Go to 5a,6b,12,14
(d) Atrial activation begins in His bundle recording lead		
• Yes	AV nodal reentrant SVT *or* Junctional ectopic tachycardia *or* SVT (or VT) conducting via intermediate septal accessory pathway *or* Antidromic SVT	Go to 5a,6b,12,14
(e) Atrial activation begins in right atrium		
• Yes	Atrial automatic SVT *or* Atrial reentrant SVT *or* SVT or VT conducting via right free wall accessory pathway	Go to 5a,6b,12,15

12. Introduction of single VPB during His bundle refractory period resets atrium during tachycardia with same atrial activation sequence as during tachycardia

   • Yes   SVT utilizing accessory pathway   Go to 15

13. Introduction of single or double APB during tachycardia resets tachycardia

   • Yes   Most supraventricular tachycardias

Table I. Diagnostic Approach to Paroxysmal Tachycardia—*(Continued)*

Question/Answer	Conclusion	Next Step
• No	AV nodal reentrant SVT *or*	Go to 5a,14
	Junctional ectopic tachycardia *or*	Go to 5c
	Ventricular tachycardia *or*	Go to 10,16,18
	Atrial flutter or fibrillation	Go to 5b

14. Initiation of SVT depends on achieving critical AH interval

   • Yes   AV nodal reentrant SVT

15. Initiation on SVT depends on achieving critical AV interval without necessarily depending on AH interval

   • Yes   Orthodromic SVT using an accessory pathway

16. Initiation and maintenance of wide-QRS tachycardia depends on critical VH interval

   • Yes   BB reentrant VT *or* Mahaim fiber tachycardia (long V-H type)

17. Initiation and maintenance of wide QRS tachycardia depends on critical VA interval without necessarily depending on VH interval

   • Yes   Antidromic SVT in WPW *or* Orthodromic SVT with BBB   Go to 9

Table I. Diagnostic Approach to Paroxysmal Tachycardia—(Continued)

Question/Answer	Conclusion	Next Step

18. During wide QRS tachycardia, atrial stimulation exactly reproduces QRS of the tachycardia during conducted atrial beats

   • Yes

> SVT with BBB or "bystander" accessory pathway Mahaim fiber tachycardias.
> (Note that after the conducted beat, QRS may become normal, with loss of BBB or bystander Mahaim or accessory pathway participation. This will then permit analysis of step 9b.)

   • No

> Ventricular tachycardia

   • Fusion beats

> Typical of VT
> Also seen with preexcited SVTs   Go to 21

19. Initiation of SVT dependent on critical A_1A_2 or A_2A_3 coupling interval without the initiating beat necessarily conducting to ventricle.

   • Yes

> Atrial reentrant SVT or AV nodal reentrant SVT   Go to 20
> (Consider this only if block occurs distal to His)

20. Initiation of SVT dependent on critical A_1A_2 or A_2A_3 coupling interval without the initiating beat necessarily conducting to His bundle.

   • Yes   Atrial reentrant SVT

21. Initiation of wide QRS tachycardia dependent on critical V_1V_2, V_2V_3 or V_3V_4 coupling interval without the initiating beat necessarily conducting to His bundle or atrium.

Table I. Diagnostic Approach to Paroxysmal Tachycardia—(Continued)

Question/Answer	Conclusion	Next Step
• Yes	Ventricular tachycardia	

22. Tachycardia not able to be initiated, reset, entrained or terminated by programmed stimulation.

• Yes	Mechanism probably other than reentrant	Consider exercise testing, isoproterenol, provocation by antiarrhythmic drugs to reproduce tachycardia

---

$A_1, A_2, A_3,$ = atrial electrograms of the spontaneous or driven atrial beats, the first paced extrastimulus, the second paced extrastimulus, respectively. APB = atrial premature beat. AH = A-H interval. AV = atrioventricular. BB = bundle branch. BBB = bundle branch block. fib = fibrillation. HPS = His-Purkinje system. HV = H-V interval. LBBB = left bundle branch block. NSR = normal sinus rhythm. PJRT = permanent form of junctional reciprocating tachycardia.[25] RBBB = right bundle branch block. RP = R-P interval. sec = seconds. SVT = supraventricular tachycardia. tach = tachycardia. $V_1 V_2 V_3 V_4$ = ventricular electrograms of the spontaneous or driven ventricular beats and of the first, second, and third paced extrastimuli, respectively. VA = ventriculoatrial V-H = V-H interval. VPB = ventricular premature beat. VT = ventricular tachycardia. WPW = Wolff-Parkinson-White syndrome.

D. Use of Bedside Maneuvers and Pharmacology in Diagnosis of Mechanism of Paroxysmal Tachycardia

Once maximum information has been obtained from passive ECG or electrogram recordings during tachycardia, it is legitimate to employ provocative vagal maneuvers and judicious use of pharmacologic agents for further information (Table II). During the course of these steps, conversion of the tachycardia may occur. Continuous ECG recording (preferably in three or more simultaneous leads) should always be performed during all such interventions. Information about mode of termination of tachycardia and about the ensuing escape rhythm can be of great diagnostic value. For example, the first sinus beat which follows a post-conversion pause may be the only beat that shows a delta wave in a patient with paroxysmal SVT due to an otherwise concealed accessory pathway.

Table II. Diagnostic Use of Bedside Maneuvers and Pharmacology

1. Explore as many steps from Table I as possible, given the prevailing constraints of the clinical situation.

2. Switch on three-channel ECG strip chart recorder and keep it running.

3. Deep tidal respiration.

- Phasic variation in rate implies tachycardia sensitive to autonomic modulation, e.g., sinus rhythm.

4. Right, then left carotid massage.

- Transient slowing of rate of tachycardia without AV block implies tachycardia sensitive to vagal activity, e.g., sinus rhythm, reentrant SVT (AV node at least one limb of the circuit). During the pause, examine P waves and return to Table I, step 4.

- Transient slowing of rate of ventricular response because of second or third degree AV block, without conversion of tachycardia, implies a

Table II. Diagnostic Use of Bedside Maneuvers and Pharmacology—(Continued)

mechanism confined to the atria, e.g., atrial reentrant or automatic SVT, atrial flutter, atrial fibrillation. During the pause in AV conduction, examine atrial activity. *Atrial flutter* is diagnosed by atrial activity that is uniform in cycle length, morphology, amplitude, and polarity and has a rate roughly between 240 and 360 per minute. *Atrial fibrillation* is diagnosed by atrial activity that is variable in cycle length, morphology, amplitude and polarity, generally with a rate in excess of 350 per minute.

- Conversion of tachycardia. Examine the last few cycles of tachycardia for P waves. Determine the presence or absence of a P wave after the last QRS. Return to Table I, step 8. Note that carotid massage frequently causes termination of tachycardias by inducing ventricular premature beats. Termination of SVT by one or more VPBs implies that either the ventricular muscle or part or all of the AV conduction system is part of the reentrant circuit. (See Table I, step 12). Atrial and AV nodal reentrant tachycardias are rarely reset by single VPBs but AV nodal reentrant SVT is frequently terminated by vagal maneuvers per se.

5. Other vagomimetic maneuvers.

- The diving reflex (elicited by facial immersion in cold water), Valsalva maneuver, Mueller's maneuver, adopting the supine posture, or excitation of the baroreceptor can all produce vagal effects in certain individuals.

- In this era, pharmacologic elevation of blood pressure (phenylephrine, metaraminol, levarterenol, etc.) is discouraged because these may lead to enhanced double product and therefore could endanger the patient already in tachycardia if they do not immediately convert the arrhythmia. Also, in VT, these measures are usually ineffective.

- Ocular pressure as a vagomimetic maneuver is to be avoided because it is painful and because it may cause ocular damage, especially in the presence of scleromalacia.

- If the patient is tolerating the tachycardia well, and it is clearly SVT, then sleep is one of the most powerful vagomimetic maneuvers and is nearly always effective.

- The interpretation of the results of these alternative maneuvers is similar to that for carotid massage.

Table II. Diagnostic Use of Bedside Maneuvers and Pharmacology—*(Continued)*

6. Use of intravenous verapamil.

- Verapamil should only be given if the mechanism of the tachycardia is clearly supraventricular. The onus is on the physician to be able to prove this unequivocally in the event of an adverse hemodynamic response to this powerful negative inotropic agent.

- The correct dose of verapamil is 0.15 mg/kg body weight over 2 minutes (10.5 mg in a 70 kg adult). Less than this may convert SVT or produce AV block in atrial flutter or fibrillation. However a negative response to this drug cannot be presumed until the full dose is administered.

- As with vagomimetic maneuvers, verapamil may cause interruption of SVT by first inducing VPBs. Diagnostic information may again be yielded.

- The post-conversion pause after verapamil may be quite long because of suppression of sinus node automaticity. For this reason, verapamil should never be given in patients with known sinus node dysfunction, without a functioning temporary or permanent pacemaker. This pause, however, may also yield important diagnostic information as noted in Table II, elsewhere.

- Emergency equipment should always be immediately available when administering any drug during a tachycardia.

7. Use of other antiarrhythmic drugs.

- In patients with SVT, short acting drugs such as esmolol or adenosine are highly efficacious in terminating or slowing tachycardias in which the AV node is involved in the reentrant circuit or in which the AV node is in control of ventricular rate.

- The use of class I antiarrhythmic drugs by the intravenous route should be reserved for situations where the mechanism of tachycardia is known, or when specific diagnostic information cannot be achieved any other way. For example, in atrial fibrillation conducting by way of an accessory pathway, intravenous procainamide or lidocaine have been used to block the accessory pathway, so slowing the ventricular

Table II. Diagnostic Use of Bedside Maneuvers and Pharmacology—(Continued)

response as well as exposing conduction via the normal AV conduction system.

8. Use of pacing techniques in diagnosis and termination of paroxysmal tachycardias.

- Table I (steps 11 through 22) summarizes the practical usefulness of pacing techniques.

- Whenever pacing is utilized, equipment for cardiac resuscitaiton should always be immediately available.

- Pacing, like cardioversion, may have increased risk in the presence of digitalis intoxication.

- Sufficient current, sufficient rate, and sufficient duration of pacing should be employed to obtain reliable capture of the chamber paced. It may be difficult to discern whether capture is occurring in the case of the atria. This is one circumstance where simultaneous atrial recording is especially helpful.

- When pacing the atrium in atrial flutter, it is generally advisable to use current in the range of 10 to 20 mA, and a duration of pacing of 10 to 60 seconds before observing for termination of atrial flutter. The reader should review the recommendations of Waldo[24] in using pacing for atrial flutter.

9. Use of DC cardioversion for paroxysmal tachycardias.

- Whenever a patient is unconscious or gravely obtunded due to a paroxysmal tachycardia, synchronized DC cardioversion should be performed without elaborate diagnostic maneuvers.

- However, even in the most emergent situations, there is always time to make a recording of the arrhythmia on a monitor strip chart recorder. There is also almost always time to record at least the six frontal plane leads from a monitor, and frequently also enough time to obtain a 12-lead ECG. The diagnostic value of this step for future therapy cannot be over emphasized.

- Unless the rhythm is ventricular fibrillation, reversion should always be performed in the synchronous mode.

Table II. Diagnostic Use of Bedside Maneuvers and Pharmacology—*(Continued)*

- Preparation for more elective cardioversion should be as for general anesthesia with proper attention to airway, ventilation, blood pressure support, intravascular volume, and preparation for cardiovascular resuscitation if it becomes necessary.

- This author prefers the use of short acting general anesthetics such as Brevital or Etomidate rather than Valium. These agents give much better anesthesia and are more reliable in terms of dose requirements in patients who might be constitutionally resistant to Valium and similar sedatives.

- Energy used for elective cardioversion should be the minimum consistent with a high likelihood of success in reversion to sinus rhythm. For PSVT, energies of 20 to 50 J are generally adequate—for atrial flutter 50 to 150 J, atrial fibrillation 100 to 300 J, ventricular tachycardia 50 to 200 J for most patients.

REFERENCES

1. Scherlag BJ, Lau SH, Helfant RM, Stein H, Berkowitz WD, Damato AN: Catheter technique for recording His bundle activity in man. *Circulation* 1969; 39:13.

2. Goldreyer BN, Damato AN: The essential role of atrioventricular conduction delay in the initiation of paroxysmal supraventricular tachycardia. *Circulation* 1971; 43:679.

3. Denes P, Wu D, Dhingra RC, Chuquimia R, Rosen KM: Demonstration of dual A-V nodal pathways in patients with paroxysmal supraventricular tachycardia. *Circulation* 1973; 48:549.

4. Wu D, Denes P, Amat-y-Leon F, Dhingra R, Wyndham CR, Bauernfeind R, Latif P, Rosen KM: Clinical, electrocardiographic and electrophysiologic observations in patients with paroxysmal supraventricular tachycardia. *Am J Cardiol* 1978; 41:1045.

5. Wellens HJJ, Schuilenburg RM, Durrer D: Electrical stimulation of the heart in patients with ventricular tachycardia. *Circulation* 1972; 46:216.

6. Wu D, Wyndham CRC, Denes P, Dhingra R, Bauernfeind R, Swiryn S, Rosen KM: Chronic electrophysiological study in patients with recurrent paroxysmal tachycardia: A new method for developing successful oral antiarrhythmic therapy. In: Kulbertus HE, ed. *Reentrant Arrhythmias.* Lancaster, England: MTP 1977; pp. 294-311.

7. Denes P, Wu D, Wyndham CRC, Dhingra R, Bauernfiend R, Swiryn S, Rosen KM: Chronic electrophysiologic study of ventricular tachycardia. *Chest* 1980; 77:478.

8. Gallagher JJ, Gilbert M, Svenson RH, Sealy WC, Kasell J, Wallace AG: Wolff-Parkinson-White syndrome: The problem, evaluation, and surgical considerations. *Circulation* 1975; 51:767.

9. Scheinman MM, Morady F, Hess DS, Gonzalez R: Catheter-induced ablation of the atrioventricular

junction to control refractory supraventricular arrhythmias. *J Am Med Assoc* 1982; 248:851.

10. den Dulk K, Bertholet M, Brugada P, Bär FW. Demoulin JC, Waleffe A, Bakels N, Lindemans F, Bourgeois I, Kulbertus HE, et al: Clinical experience with implantable devices for control of tachyarrhythmias. *PACE* 1984; 7:548.

11. Mirowski M, Reid PR, Mower MM, Watkins L, Gott VL, Schauble JF, Langer A, Heilman MS, Kolenik SA, Fischell RE, Weisfeldt ML: Termination of malignant ventricular arrhythmias with an implantable automatic defibrillator in human beings. *N Engl J Med* 1980; 303:322.

12. Dhingra RC, Rosen KM, Rahimtoola SH: Normal conduction intervals and responses in 61 patients using His bundle recording and atrial pacing. *Chest* 1973; 64:55.

13. Denes P, Wu D, Dhingra R, Pietras RJ, Rosen KM: The effects of cycle length on cardiac refractory periods in man. *Circulation* 1974; 49:32.

14. Rosen KM, Rahimtoola SH, Gunnar RM: Site and type of second degree A-V block. *Chest* 1972; 51:99.

15. Ross DL, Johnson DC, Denniss AR, Cooper MJ, Richards DA, Uther JB: Curative surgery for atrioventricular junctional ("A-V nodal") reentrant tachycardia. *J Am Coll Cardiol* 1985; 6:1383.

16. Bär FW, Brugada P, Dassen WRM, Wellens HJJ: Differential diagnosis of tachycardia with narrow QRS complex (shorter than 0.12 second). *Am J Cardiol* 1984; 54:555.

17. Wu D, Amat-y-Leon F, Denes P, Dhingra RC, Pietras RJ, Rosen KM: Demonstration of sustained sinus and atrial reentry as a mechanism of paroxysmal supraventricular tachycardia. *Circulation* 1975; 51:234.

18. Bauernfeind RA, Wyndham CRC, Dhingra RC, Swiryn SP, Palileo E, Strasberg B, Rosen KM: Serial electrophysiologic testing of multiple drugs in pa-

tients with atrioventricular nodal reentrant paroxysmal tachycardia. *Circulation* 1980; 62:1341.

19. Mann DE, Reiter MR: Effects of upright posture on atrioventricular nodal reentry and dual atrioventricular nodal pathways. *Am J Cardiol* 1988; 62:408-412.

20. Marriott HJL, Sandler IA: Criteria, old and new, for differentiating between ectopic ventricular beats and aberrant ventricular conduction in the presence of atrial fibrillation. *Prog Cardiovasc Dis* 1966; 9:18.

21. Wellens HJJ, Bär FHWM, Lie KI: The value of the electrocardiogram in the differential diagnosis of a tachycardia with a widened QRS complex. *Am J Med* 1978; 64:27.

22. Akhtar M: Electrophysiologic bases for wide QRS complex tachycardia. *PACE* 1983; 6:81.

23. Benditt DG, Pritchett ELC, Gallagher JJ: Spectrum of regular tachycardias with wide QRS complexes in patients with accessory atrioventricular pathways. *Am J Cardiol* 1978; 42:828.

24. Waldo AL, MacLean WAH, Karp RB, Kouchoukos NT, James TN: Entrainment and interruption of atrial flutter with atrial pacing: Studies in man following open-heart surgery. *Circulation* 1977; 56:737.

25. Gallagher JJ, Sealy WC: The permanent form of junctional reciprocating tachycardia: Further elucidation of the underlying mechanism. *Eur J Cardiol* 1978; 8:413.

26. Ellenbogen KA, Ramirez NM, Packer DL, O'Collaghan WG, Greer GS, Sintetos AL, Gilbert MR, German LD: Accessory nodoventricular (Mahaim) fibers: a clinical review. *PACE* 1986; 9:868.

APPENDIX A

Abbreviations for Figures

1, 11, 111, V_1: surface ECG leads 1, 11, 111, V_1
ra: right atrial electrogram
raa: right atrial appendage electrogram
lsra: low septal right atrial electrogram
hb: His bundle electrogram
cso: coronary sinus orifice electrogram
cs1, cs2, cs3, cs4, etc : electrograms 1, 2, 3, 4, etc., cms inside cso
rva: right ventricular apex electrogram
A: atrial electrogram
H: His bundle deflection
msec: milliseconds
CL: cycle length (in msec)
a-h: A-H interval (in msec)
VA: ventriculo-atrial interval (in msec)
h-v: HV interval (in msec)
PAT: paroxysmal atrial tachycardia
NSR: normal sinus rhythm
VT: ventricular tachycardia
⋏ : retrograde block
⋎ : anterograde block
ឋ : pacing stimulus
✱ : datum line drawn to define onset of QRS

APPENDIX B

Cycle Length (msec) $\times$ Rate (bpm) $= 60,000$

CL	HR	CL	HR	CL	HR
50	1,200	320	188	590	102
100	600	330	181	600	100
109	550	333	180	620	97
120	500	340	176	640	94
133	450	350	171	660	91
150	400	353	170	667	90
160	375	360	167	680	88
170	353	370	162	700	86
171	350	375	160	750	80
180	333	380	158	800	75
190	316	390	154	850	71
200	300	400	150	857	70
207	290	410	146	900	67
210	286	420	143	950	63
214	280	430	140	1,000	60
220	273	440	136	1,050	57
222	270	450	133	1,100	55
230	261	460	130	1,150	52
231	260	470	128	1,200	50
240	250	480	125	1,300	46
250	240	490	122	1,400	43
260	231	500	120	1,500	40
261	230	510	118	1,600	38
270	222	520	115	1,700	35
273	220	530	113	1,800	33
280	214	540	111	1,900	32
286	210	''45	110	2,000	30
290	207	550	109	2,400	25
300	200	560	107	2,500	24
310	193	570	105	3,000	20
316	190	580	103		

In keeping with the style of a programmed text, several clinical examples of paroxysmal tachycardias are presented in a quiz-like format. The reader should study the electrocardiograms carefully, utilizing the foregoing approach, arrive at a probable diagnosis, then refer to the author's interpretation for confirmation. The mechanism of tachycardia was confirmed by catheter electrophysiologic techniques in each case.

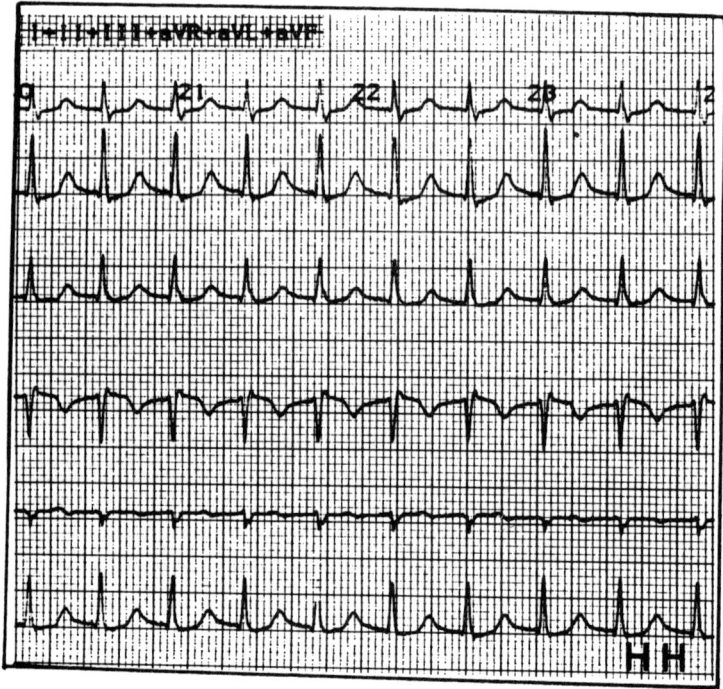

Figure 1A. 25-Year-Old Female

Cycle length (msec):
Rate (bpm):
QRS duration (msec):
Regularity; Yes/No
    Group Beating?
P waves visible? Yes/No
P waves associated? Yes/No
    If so, long or short R-P?
    P wave vector:
Describe QRS morphology: V_1____V_6____
QRS axis:

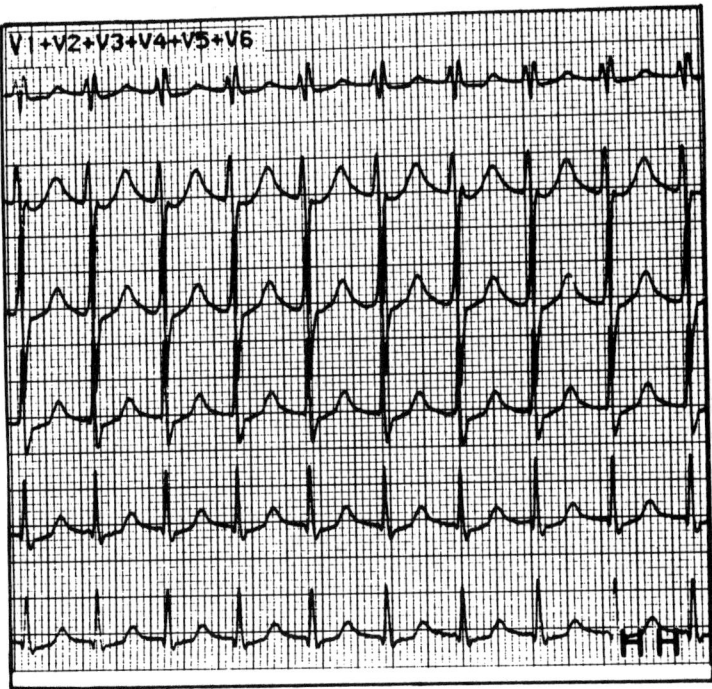

Figure 1B. No Heart Disease

Probable arrhythmia diagnosis: _____

   If SVT, probable mechanism: _____

   If VT, probable site of origin: _____

Next diagnostic maneuver:

1. Vagal maneuver   [ ]
2. Atrial or esophageal electrogram   [ ]
3. Administration of verapamil, esmolol or adenosine   [ ]
4. Administration of lidocaine or procainamide   [ ]
5. Administration of atropine or isoproterenol   [ ]
6. Synchronized DC cardioversion   [ ]
7. His bundle recording   [ ]
8. Programmed stimulation   [ ]

Paroxysmal Atrioventricular Nodal Reentrant Tachycardia
Cycle length: 390 msec
Rate: 154 bpm
QRS: 90 msec
Regular
P waves are not apparent at first glance but are actually inscribed
in the terminal QRS producing a "pseudo-R-prime" in leads V_1
and aVR.

QRS morphology: Constant (no alternans) and appears to show
incomplete RBBB. Only comparison with the ECG in sinus rhythm
will determine whether terminal RV conduction delay or a superimposed retrograde P wave is the cause of this terminal QRS
vector.

QRS axis: 65°

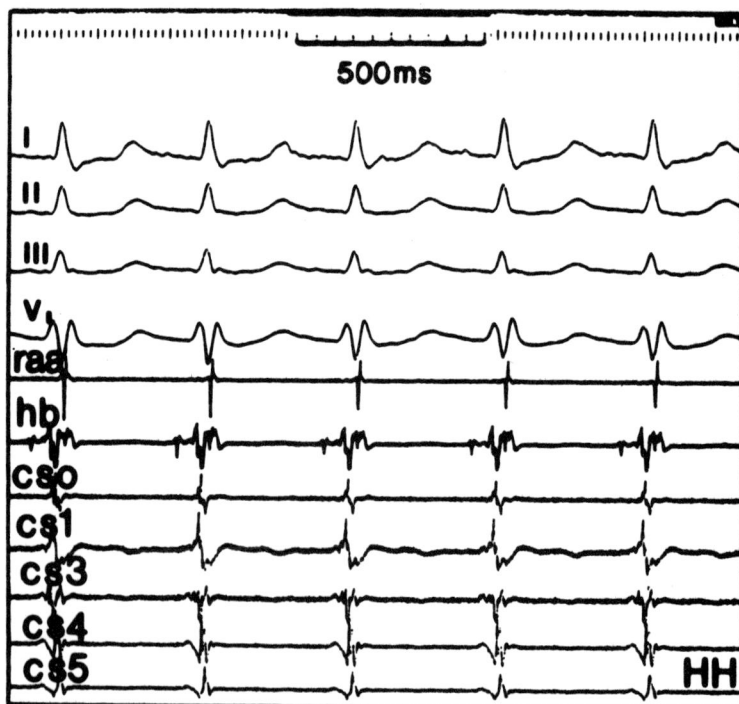

Figure 1C.

Comment:

The retrograde P wave of atrioventricular nodal reentrant SVT is typically inscribed at this time in the cardiac cycle, simultaneously with the QRS (see intracardiac recording in Figure 1C) [Table I, step 4,5]. This is because the H-A interval on the retrograde fast atrioventricular nodal pathway is similar to the H-V interval. At the bedside, with a strip chart recorder running, carotid sinus massage or other vagal maneuvers may slow or interrupt the SVT. The absence of the deflection representing the retrograde P wave during sinus rhythm will readily permit an initial diagnosis of atrioventricular nodal reentrant SVT (see isolated sinus beat in Figure 1D). Note, during SVT (Figure 1C), the retrograde P wave vector is oriented forward and somewhat inferiorly consistent with initial atrial activation in the mid-septum. In the intracardiac recordings, atrial activity is first detected in the His bundle recording lead a little before that in the coronary sinus orifice and more leftward sites in the coronary sinus [Table I, step 11].

Abbreviations: Appendix A.

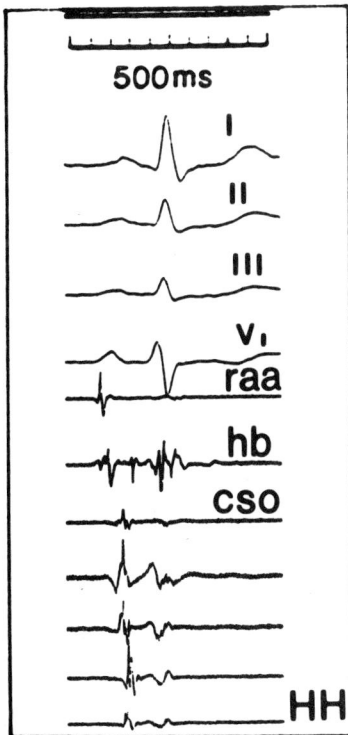

Figure 1D.

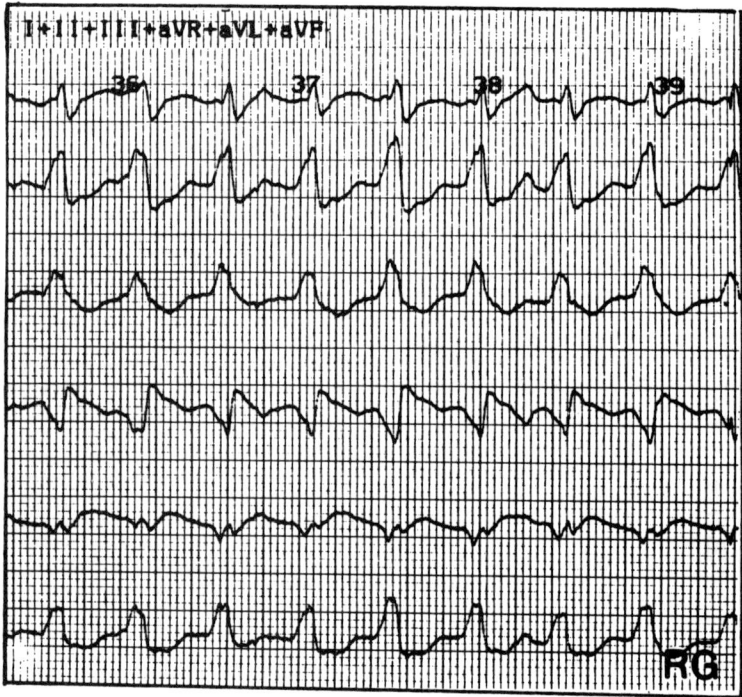

Figure 2A. 75-Year-Old Male

Cycle length (msec):
Rate (bpm):
QRS duration (msec):
Regularity; Yes/No
  Group Beating?
P waves visible? Yes/No
P waves associated? Yes/No
  If so, long or short R-P?
  P wave vector:
Describe QRS morphology: V₁——— V₆———
QRS axis:

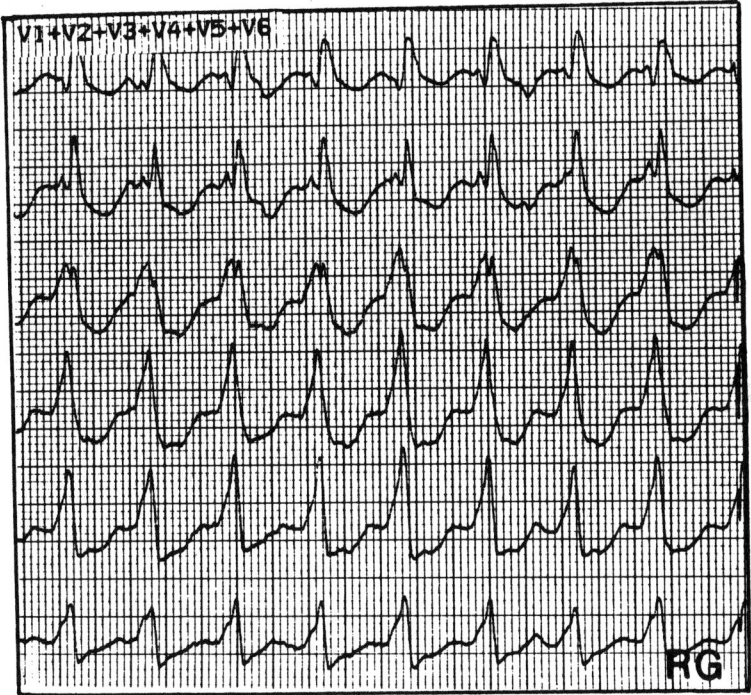

Figure 2B. Previous Myocardial Infarction.

Probable arrhythmia diagnosis: _____
    If SVT, probable mechanism: _____
    If VT, probable site of origin: _____
Next diagnostic maneuver:
1. Vagal maneuver   [ ]
2. Atrial or esophageal   [ ]
electrogram
3 Administration of verapamil,
    esmolol or adenosine   [ ]
4. Administration of lidocaine or
    procainamide   [ ]
5. Administration of atropine or
    isoproterenol   [ ]
6. Synchronized DC cardioversion   [ ]
7. His bundle recording   [ ]
8. Programmed stimulation   [ ]

Sustained Ventricular Tachycardia.
Cycle length: 460 msec
Rate: 130 bpm
QRS: 200 msec
Regular
P waves visible and dissociated.
QRS morphology: rsR in V_1, Rs in V_6
QRS axis: 105°

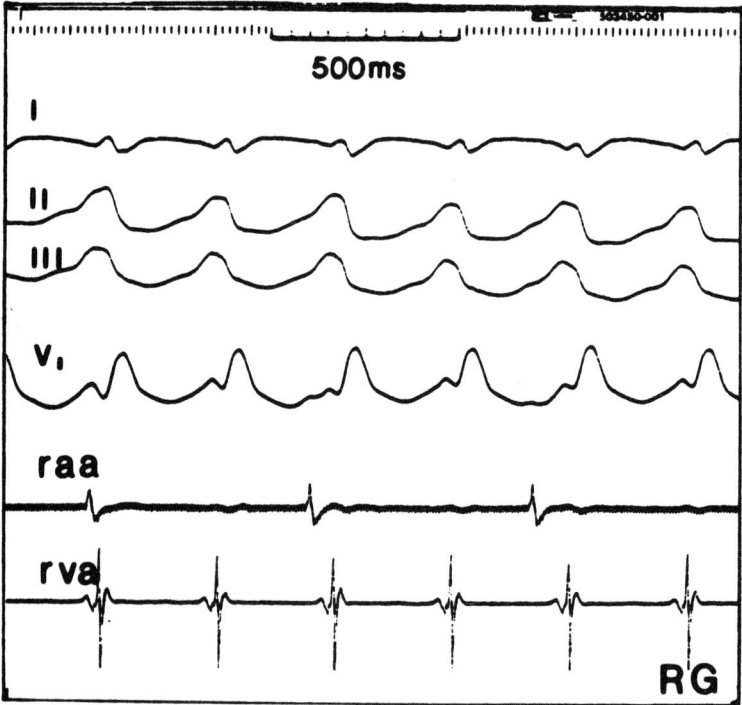

Figure 2C.

Comment:
Note atrioventricular dissociation, best seen in leads II, aVR, V_2 and V_6, confirming the diagnosis of VT in presence of very wide QRS and abnormal frontal plane axis [Table I, step 5]. The small initial R wave in V_2 resembles a P wave but is clearly part of the QRS if its timing is compared to the onset of QRS in other leads. The initial QRS vector is directed forward, downward, leftward and toward the cardiac apex (V_6) suggesting an initial site of ventricular activation in the basal anterior left ventricular wall. The atrial electrogram recorded at another time (Figure 2C) shows a 2 :1 ventriculoatrial relationship suggesting retrograde capture of the atria. Some ventriculoatrial conduction is apparent in about 50% of cases of ventricular tachycardia. However, careful measurement in this case shows that the ventriculoatrial interval progressively shortens, indicating atrioventricular dissociation.

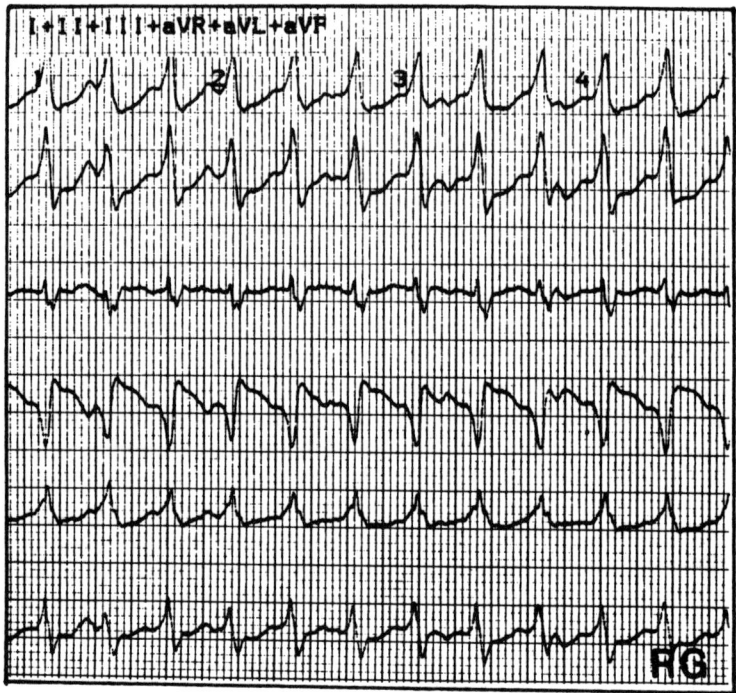

Figure 3A. 75-Year-Old Male.

Cycle length (msec): _____
Rate (bpm): _____
QRS duration (msec): _____
Regularity; Yes/No _____
  Group Beating? _____
P waves visible? Yes/No _____
P waves associated? Yes/No _____
  If so, long or short R-P? _____
  P wave vector: _____
Describe QRS morphology: V_1—V_6—
QRS axis: _____

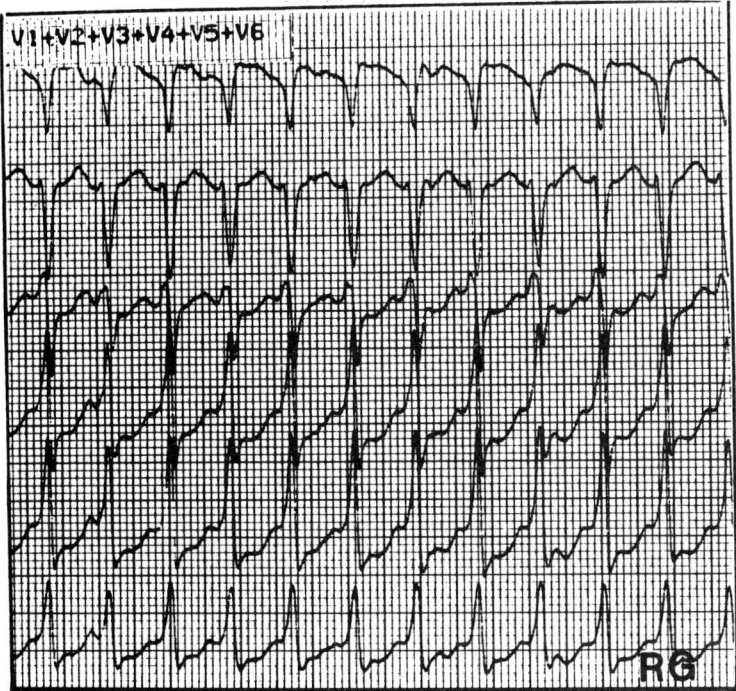

Figure 3B. Previous Myocardial Infarction.

Probable arrhythmia diagnosis: _____
   If SVT, probable mechanism: _____
   If VT, probable site of origin: _____
Next diagnostic maneuver:
  1. Vagal maneuver   [ ]
  2. Atrial or esophageal electrogram   [ ]
  3. Administration of verapamil, esmolol or
     adenosine   [ ]
  4. Administration of lidocaine or procainamide   [ ]
  5. Administration of atropine or isoproterenol   [ ]
  6. Synchronized DC cardioversion   [ ]
  7. His bundle recording   [ ]
  8. Programmed stimulation   [ ]

Sustained Ventricular Tachycardia
Cycle length: 350 msec
Rate: 171 bpm
QRS: 140 msec
Regular
P waves visible and dissociated.
QRS morphology: Qr in V_1; Rs in V_6
QRS axis: $-20°$

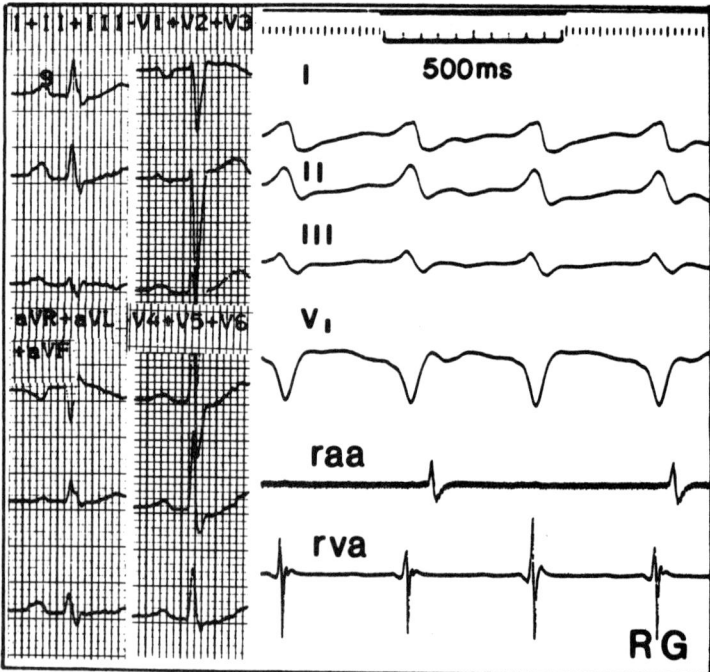

Figure 3C.

Comment:

Note atrioventricular dissociation, best seen in leads II, aVR, V_1 [Table I, step 5]. This confirms VT despite the borderline wide QRS, normal frontal plane axis and largely upright QRS in V_6 [Table I, step 1, 10]. Atrioventricular dissociation was proven by atrial recording shown in Figure 3C. Initial QRS vector is oriented posteriorly, leftward, horizontally and somewhat toward the cardiac apex (V_6), suggesting a site of earliest ventricular activation near the basal, anterior septum or right ventricle. In both the tachycardias in this patient (#2, #3) the Q wave in V_1 is a Q wave that "remembers" the site of infarction. The anterior infarction was not associated with residual Q waves in the ECG during sinus rhythm as shown in Figure 3C. Since the tachycardias most likely emanated from the septal border zone, the initial forces of the QRS during tachycardia resemble the Q waves of the previous infarct.

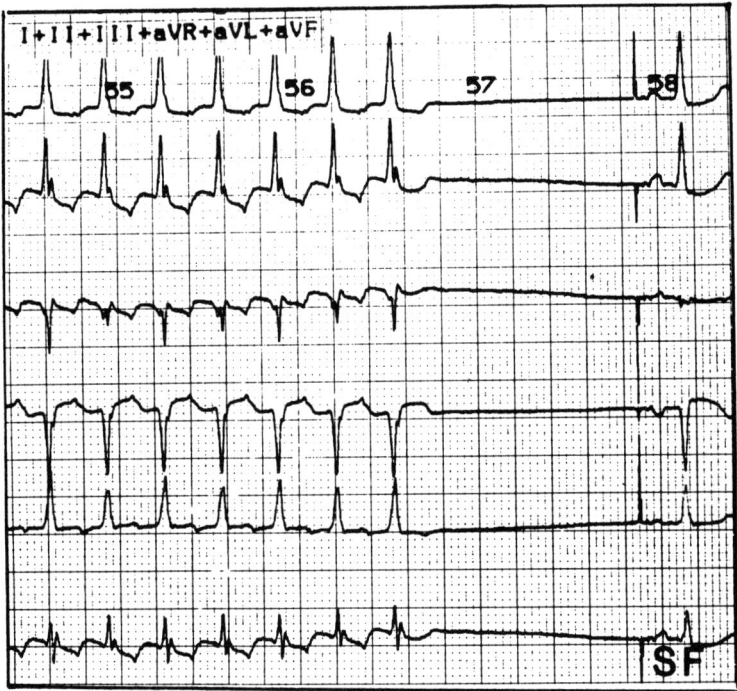

Figure 4A. 34-Year-Old Male.

Cycle length (msec): _____
Rate (bpm): _____
QRS duration (msec): _____
Regularity; Yes/No _____
  Group Beating? _____
P waves visible? Yes/No _____
P waves associated? Yes/No _____
  If so, long or short R-P? _____
  P wave vector: _____
Describe QRS morphology: V₁—V₆—
QRS axis: _____

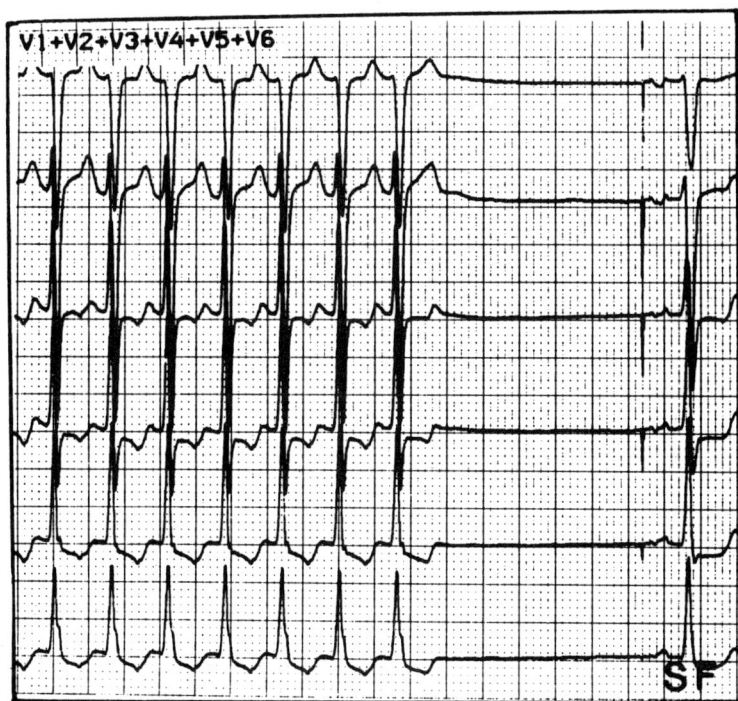

Figure 4B. No Heart Disease..

Probable arrhythmia diagnosis: _____

   If SVT, probable mechanism: _____

   If VT, probable site of origin: _____

Next diagnostic maneuver:

1. Vagal maneuver   [ ]
2. Atrial or esophageal electrogram   [ ]
3. Administration of verapamil, esmolol or
   adenosine   [ ]
4. Administration of lidocaine or procainamide   [ ]
5. Administration of atropine or isoproterenol   [ ]
6. Synchronized DC cardioversion   [ ]
7. His bundle recording   [ ]
8. Programmed stimulation   [ ]

Atrial Focal Tachycardia with Sinus Node Dysfunction
Cycle length: 330 msec
Rate: 182 bpm
Regular
P waves visible, associated with QRS.
R-P = P-R.
P wave vector rightward anterior and superior [Table I, step 4].
QRS morphology: normal
QRS axis: 10°

Comment:
The helpful features during the tachycardia in this case include the P wave morphology and the mode of termination of tachycardia. One presumes a 1:1 atrioventricular relationship during this tachycardia; however a second P wave obscured within the QRS complex cannot be excluded. If this were present, atrial flutter would be presumed and the atrial cycle length would be rather short for classical atrial flutter: 165 msec [Table I, step 5]. Therefore atrial tachycardia with 1:1 atrioventricular relationship is more likely. The termination of tachycardia shows that the QRS complex was the last tachycardia event, that is, there is no P wave following the last QRS [Table I, step 8]. These features do not allow a definitive diagnosis from the electrocardiogram alone. The differential diagnosis includes, (1) atrial focal tachycardia with 1:1 atrioventricular conduction, (2) reciprocating tachycardia utilizing an accessory pathway in which the accessory pathway is the site of block resulting in termination of tachycardia, (3) atrioventricular nodal reentrant tachycardia in which the retrograde pathway has a longer conduction time than the anterograde pathway, i.e. the so called "unusual variety" of atrioventricular nodal reentry, (4) the "permanent" form of junctional reciprocating tachycardia utilizing a slowly conducting posterior-septal accessory pathway. The absence of a P wave following the last QRS of the tachycardia effectively excludes junctional ectopic focus tachycardia with 1:1 retrograde conduction. The presence of sinus node dysfunction requiring backup demand atrial pacing implies the presence of

atrial disease and somewhat supports the diagnosis of atrial focal tachycardia. Further diagnostic studies are indicated to elucidate the mechanism of tachycardia.

The reader should inspect Figures 4C and 4D from the same patient in which the same tachycardia as the foregoing is compared with sinus rhythm.

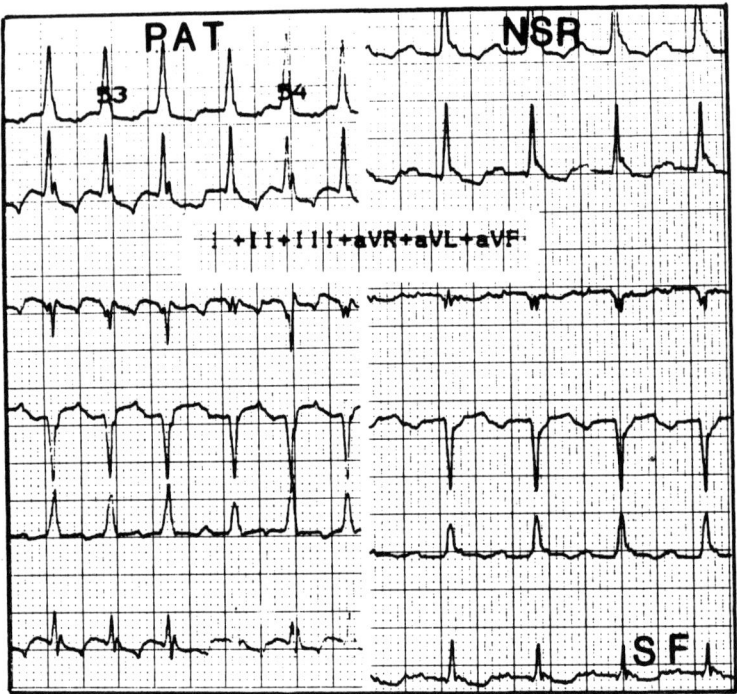

Figure 4C

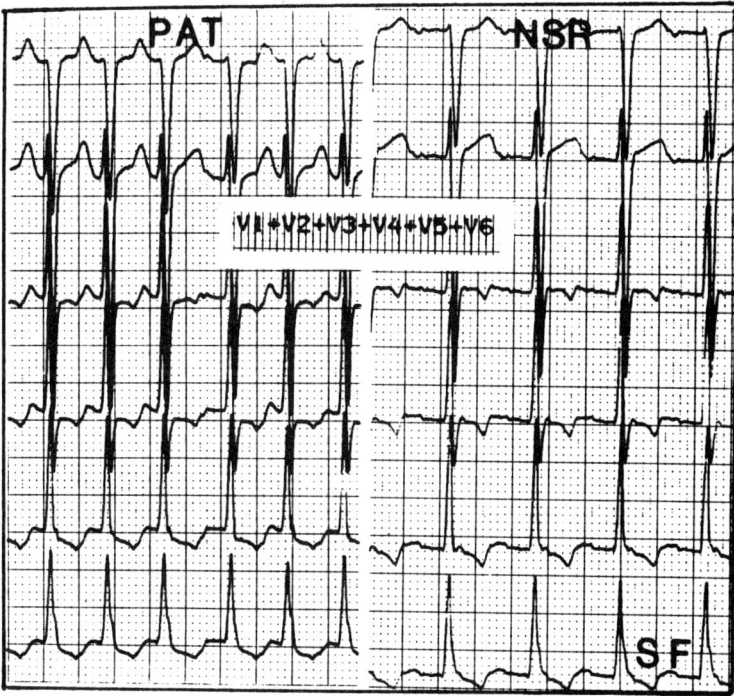

Figure 4D.

Comment:

During atrial tachycardia a brief pause occurred after the third QRS complex. Careful inspection of the timing and morphology of the P wave during this pause indicates that the QRS was late *because* the P wave was late. This finding is most consistent with atrial focal tachycardia [Table I, step 13], and is consistent with the mode of termination of tachycardia in Figures 4A and 4B in which the terminal event was the QRS.

In Figures 4C and 4D the brief pause in the tachycardia also allows further inspection of the P wave which moved off the preceding T wave sufficiently to see more clearly the P wave morphology during tachycardia. The P wave is clearly inscribed upright in V_1 during the pause. During other beats of the tachycardia the upright P wave is superimposed on the preceding T wave resulting in the T waves being somewhat more peaked. Comparison of the P wave morphology with that of sinus rhythm in the right half of each panel further demonstrates the abnormal morphology of the tachycardia P waves. Intracardiac mapping during tachycardia in this case demonstrated initial activation in the atrial septum posterior to the His bundle [Table I, step 11e].

Intracardiac recordings are shown in Figure 4E. In panel A, the mode of termination of tachycardia is demonstrated with atrial electrograms preceding QRS complexes but not following the last QRS. In panel B, a period of 2 :1 atrioventricular conduction is documented emphasizing the intraatrial mechanism of this tachycardia and the lack of dependence upon anterograde atrioventricular conduction [Table I, step 19, 20]. For practical purposes this excludes an atrioventricular reciprocating tachycardia utilizing an accessory pathway. Except in rare instances of anterograde block distal to the His bundle recording site, this finding also, in practice, excludes atrioventricular nodal reentrant tachycardia.

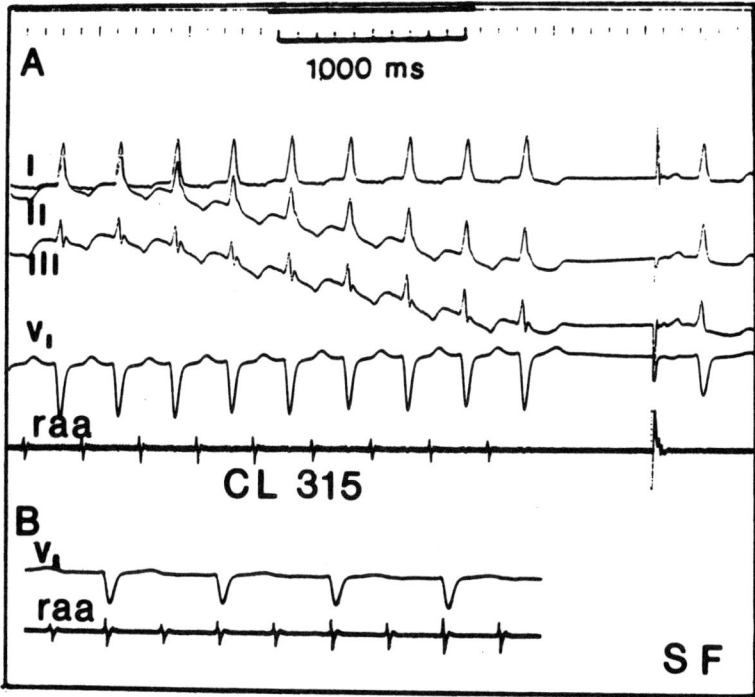

Figure 4E.

Because of the sinus node dysfunction and the occurrence of atrial flutter as a second arrhythmia in this patient, he underwent ablation of the atrioventricular conduction system and implantation of a permanent rate adaptive ventricular pacemaker.

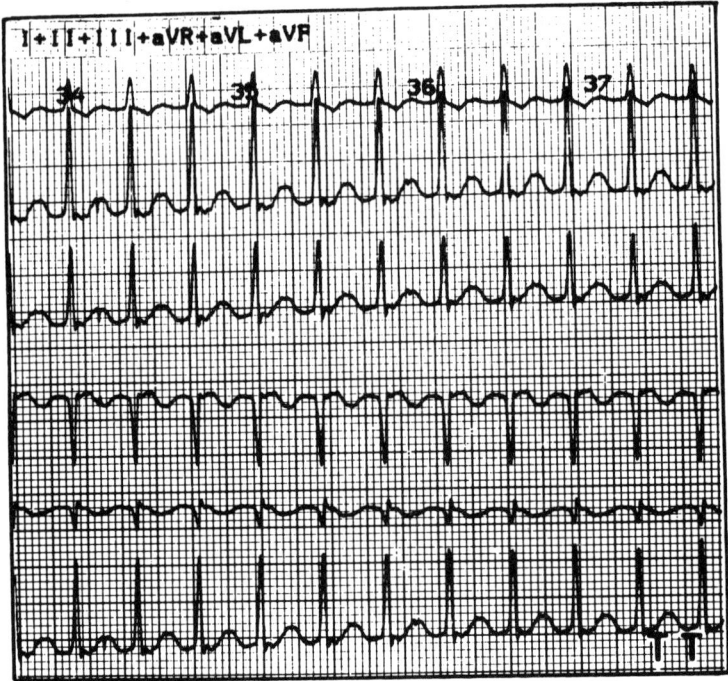

Figure 5A. 29-Year-Old Male.

Cycle length (msec):   _____
Rate (bpm):   _____
QRS duration (msec):   _____
Regularity; Yes/No   _____
   Group Beating?   _____
P waves visible? Yes/No   _____
P waves associated? Yes/No   _____
   If so, long or short R-P?   _____
   P wave vector: _____
Describe QRS morphology: V_1—V_6—
QRS axis: _____

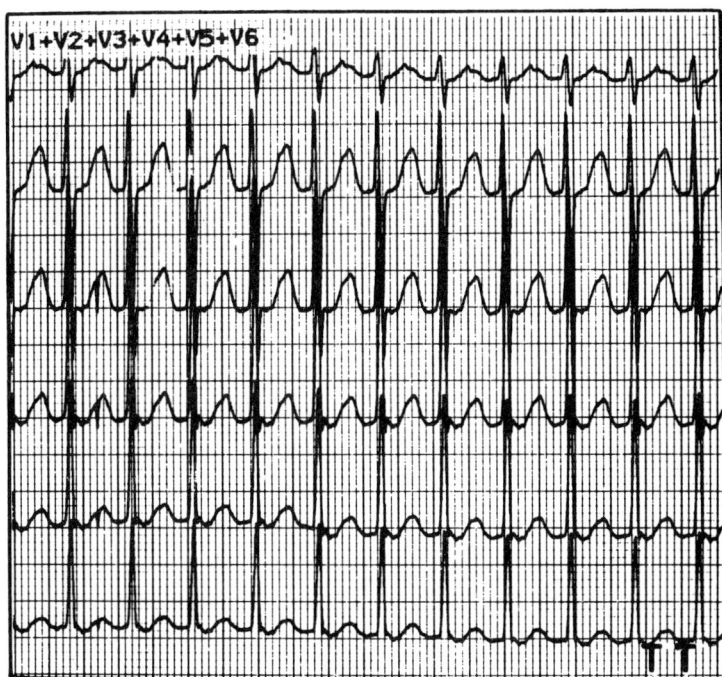

Figure 5B. No Heart Disease.

Probable arrhythmia diagnosis: _____
   If SVT, probable mechanism: _____
   If VT, probable site of origin: _____
Next diagnostic maneuver:
1. Vagal maneuver   [   ]
2. Atrial or esophageal electrogram   [   ]
3. Administration of verapamil, esmolol or
   adenosine   [   ]
4. Administration of lidocaine or procainamide   [   ]
5. Administration of atropine or isoproterenol   [   ]
6. Synchronized DC cardioversion   [   ]
7. His bundle recording   [   ]
8. Programmed stimulation   [   ]

Orthodromic Reciprocating Tachycardia
Cycle length: 355 msec
Rate: 169 bpm
QRS: 70 msec
Regular
P waves visible with major deflection approximately 120 msec after the QRS onset during the ST segment [Table I, step 5]. P wave vector is oriented rightward, anteriorly and superiorly, being negative in I, II, III, aVL, aVF, and V_3 through V_6 and positive in aVR and V_1 [Table I, step 4]. This strongly suggests the presence of a left sided accessory pathway being responsible for retrograde conduction during reciprocating tachycardia. Thus the mechanism of tachycardia is likely to be orthodromic reciprocating tachycardia utilizing a left free wall accessory pathway.
QRS axis: 70°

Comment:

The 12-lead electrocardiogram during supraventricular tachycardia contains enormous information that would not be gained from a single lead rhythm strip. The intracardiac recordings shown in Figure 5C. during reciprocating tachycardia demonstrate atrial activation initially recorded in the coronary sinus 5 cm within the coronary sinus orifice indicating the location of the atrial input from the accessory pathway to be at least this distance from the septum around the mitral annulus [Table I, step 11]. The ECG during sinus rhythm shown in Figure 5D. demonstrates Wolff-Parkinson-White Syndrome with delta wave forces oriented rightward, anteriorly and inferiorly consistent with the left free wall accessory pathway.

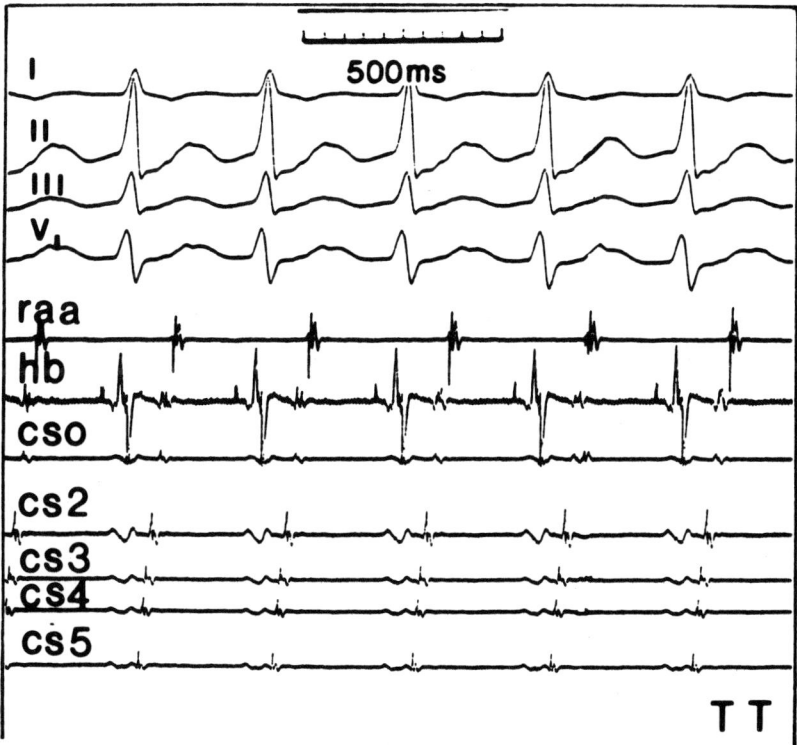

Figure 5C.

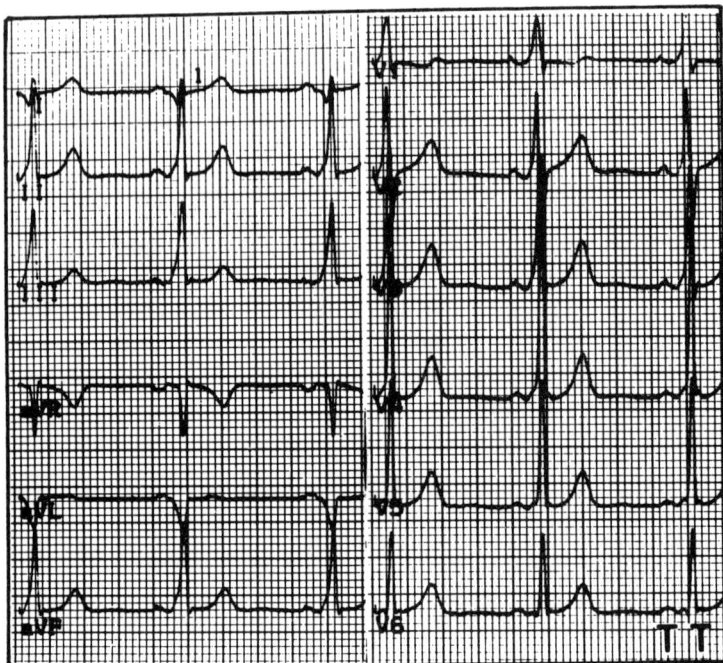

Figure 5D.

During supraventricular tachycardia vagal maneuvers may slow or interrupt the tachycardia since the atrioventricular node is an essential link in the tachycardia circuit. Following termination of tachycardia by vagal maneuvers or intravenous adenosine, verapamil or esmolol, careful inspection of the first sinus beat after conversion should show a well marked delta wave. Conversion is sometimes followed by junctional escape. If so, the QRS will be narrow without a delta wave. This is useful for comparison with subsequent preexcited beats, especially if the delta waves are more subtle than in this case. This initial vector of a junctional escape beat will generally be a fast inscription permitting identification of subtle delta waves during subsequent sinus beats.

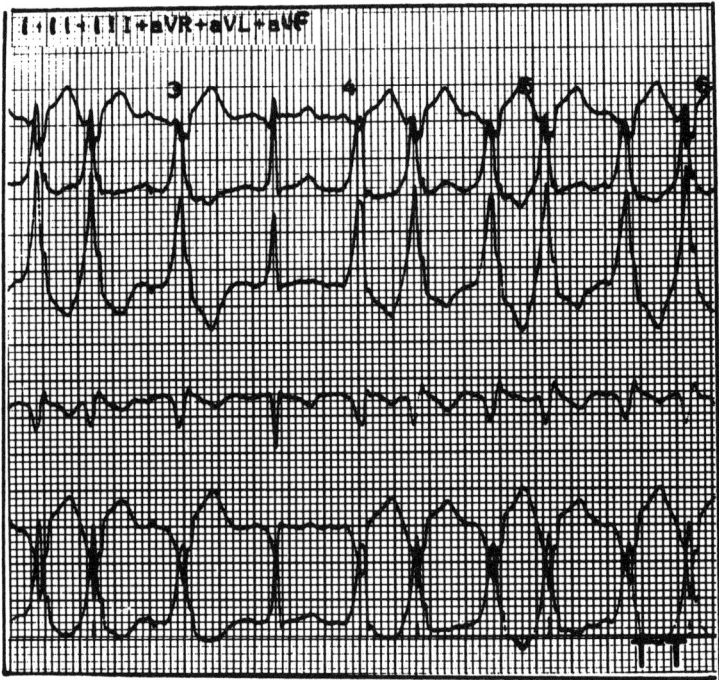

Figure 6A. 29-Year-Old Male.

Cycle length (msec):   _____

Rate (bpm):   _____

QRS duration (msec):   _____

Regularity; Yes/No   _____

   Group Beating?   _____

P waves visible? Yes/No   _____

P waves associated? Yes/No   _____

   If so, long or short R-P?   _____

   P wave vector: _____

Describe QRS morphology: V_1—V_6—

QRS axis: _____

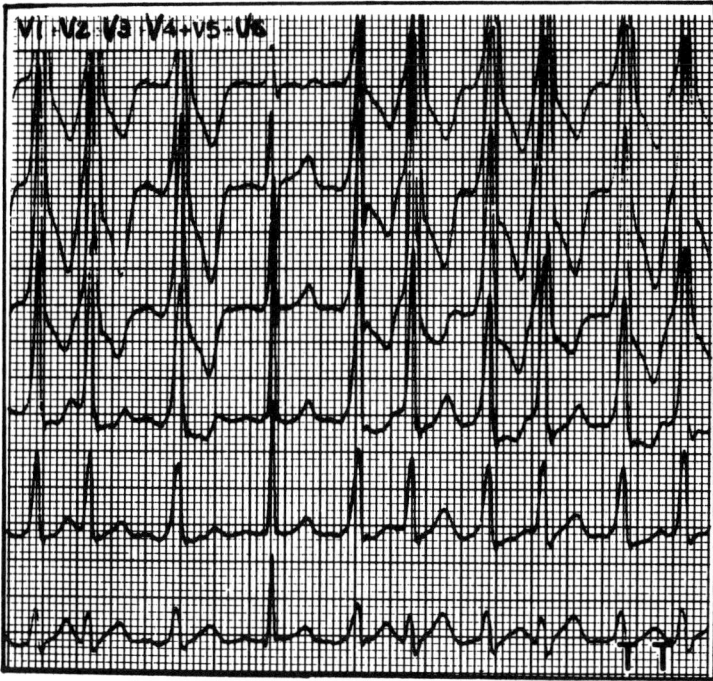

Figure 6B. No Heart Disease.

Probable arrhythmia diagnosis: _____
    If SVT, probable mechanism: _____
    If VT, probable site of origin: _____
Next diagnostic maneuver:
1. Vagal maneuver   [ ]
2. Atrial or esophageal electrogram   [ ]
3. Administration of verapamil, esmolol or
   adenosine   [ ]
4. Administration of lidocaine or procainamide   [ ]
5. Administration of atropine or isoproterenol   [ ]
6. Synchronized DC cardioversion   [ ]
7. His bundle recording   [ ]
8. Programmed stimulation   [ ]

Atrial Fibrillation, Wolff-Parkinson-White Syndrome
Cycle length: 310 to 550 msec
Rate: 109 to 194 bpm
QRS: Variable, 90 to 160 msec
Irregular
P waves not visible.
QRS morphology: Predominantly wide QRS complexes with slowing of the initial forces which are oriented rightward, anteriorly and inferiorly. One complex is relatively narrow suggesting ventricular fusion.
QRS axis: 110°

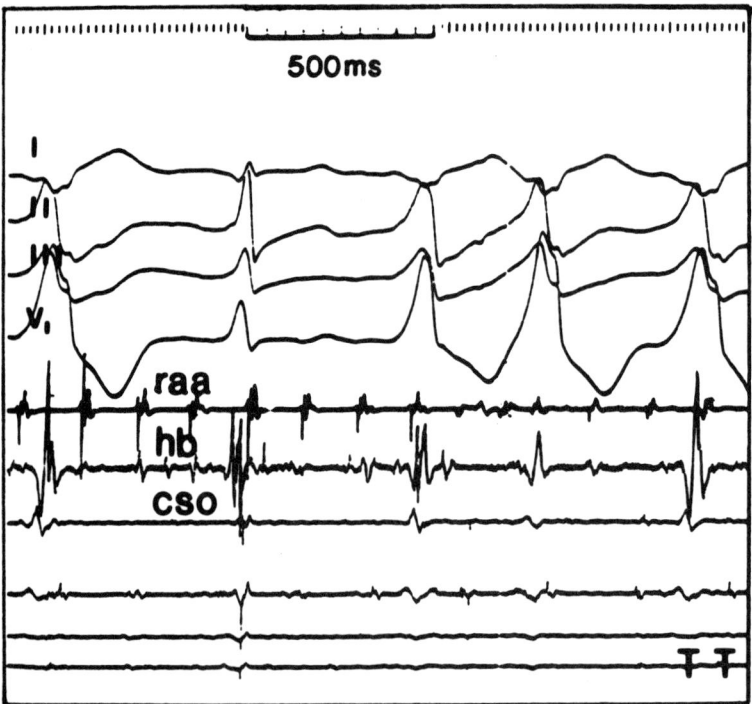

Figure 6C.

Comment:

Atrial fibrillation is diagnosed in patients with preexcitation by finding a chaotically irregular ventricular response with wide QRS resembling the delta waves of sinus rhythm. Sporadic normal pathway conduction can result in fusions or captures with normal QRS, as an isolated beat or as a short run of normal QRS complexes. Atrial fibrillation is indeed visible in the baseline in this tracing best seen in leads I, aVL and V_1 [Table II, step 4]. The ventricular response via the accessory pathway is governed by the anterograde accessory pathway refractory period; the shortest preexcited R-R interval in this case was 310 msec during this short sample. The measured anterograde refractory period in this patient was 180 msec at a cycle length of 500 msec. The intracardiac recordings shown in Figure 6C demonstrate the presence of atrial fibrillation and were recorded at the same time as the 12-lead electrocardiogram. The fusion beat seen in the 12-lead electrocardiogram is the second beat of the recording in Figure 6B. A small His bundle deflection is seen preceding this QRS.

Acute management of rapidly conducted atrial fibrillation in a patient with Wolff-Parkinson-White Syndrome will be determined by the clinical status of the patient. If the patient is severely hypotensive or obtunded, synchronized cardioversion under general anesthesia is the treatment of choice. This may also be the preferred treatment in patients who are alert and well perfused. Some authors have advocated the use of intravenous procainamide or lidocaine (Table II, 7). These drugs have the potential for further prolonging refractoriness in the accessory pathway; this effect will predictably slow the ventricular response via the accessory pathway and produce a greater proportion of normally conducted beats. One deleterious effect to be aware of is that procainamide, in slowing the atrial cycle length during atrial fibrillation and sometimes converting atrial fibrillation to atrial flutter, may have the paradoxical effect of increasing the ventricular response because of a withdrawal of the effects of repetitive anterograde concealed conduction in the accessory pathway. This may result in a paradoxical increase in heart rate. In the author's experience, one such patient then developed ventricular fibrillation and required emergency defibrillation after procainamide.

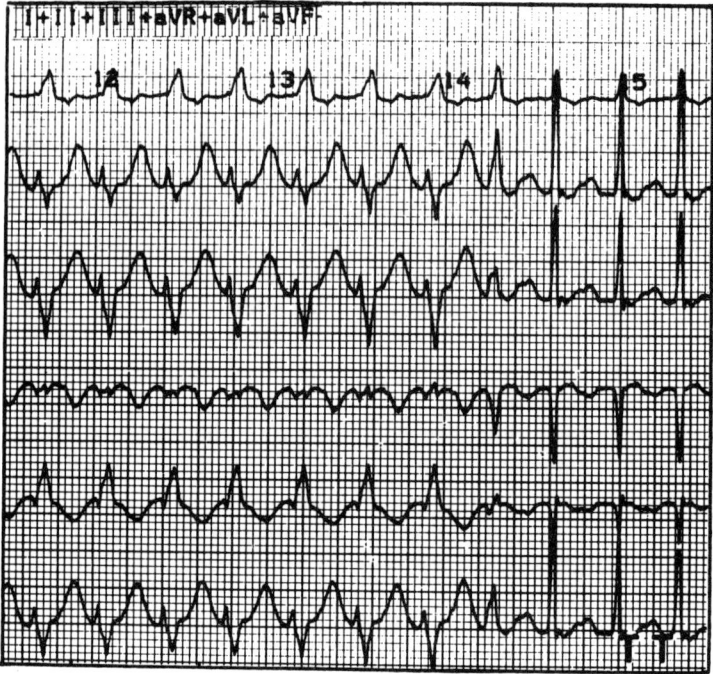

Figure 7A. 29-Year-Old Male.

Cycle length (msec): _____
Rate (bpm): _____
QRS duration (msec): _____
Regularity; Yes/No _____
  Group Beating? _____
P waves visible? Yes/No _____
P waves associated? Yes/No _____
  If so, long or short R-P? _____
  P wave vector: _____
Describe QRS morphology: V₁—V₆—
QRS axis: _____

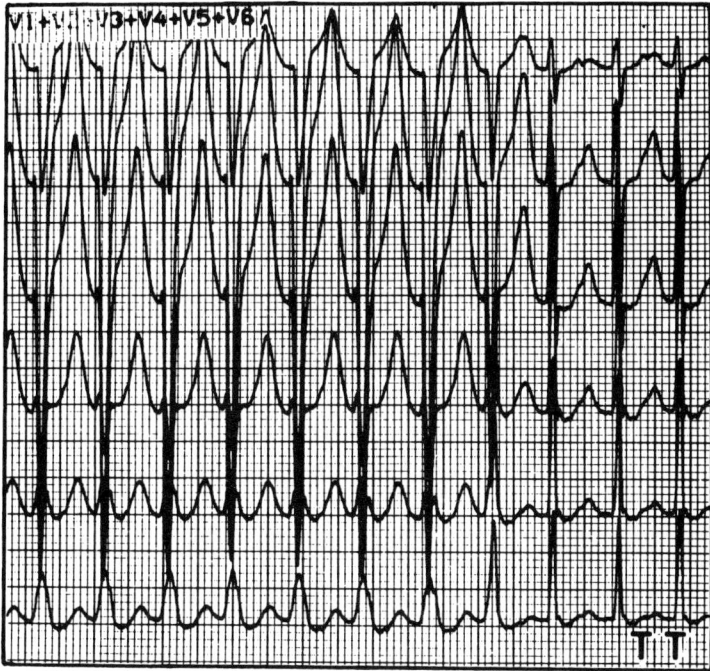

Figure 7B. No Heart Disease.

Probable arrhythmia diagnosis: _____
  If SVT, probable mechanism: _____
  If VT, probable site of origin: _____
Next diagnostic maneuver:
1. Vagal maneuver   [ ]
2. Atrial or esophageal electrogram   [ ]
3. Administration of verapamil, esmolol or
   adenosine   [ ]
4. Administration of lidocaine or procainamide [ ]
5. Administration of atropine or isoproterenol [ ]
6. Synchronized DC cardioversion   [ ]
7. His bundle recording   [ ]
8. Programmed stimulation   [ ]

Orthodromic Reciprocating Tachycardia with Left Bundle-Branch Block

Cycle length: 380 decreasing to 350 msec
Rate: 158 increasing to 171 bpm
QRS: 110 decreasing to 70 msec
Regular
P waves visible following the last three QRS complexes. P wave vector oriented rightward, superiorly and anteriorly.
QRS morphology: Left bundle-branch block during the first seven complexes [Table I, step 9e]. The eighth complex is slightly narrower, representing incomplete left bundle-branch block. The last three complexes have normal QRS configuration.
QRS axis: $-45°$ shifting to $+75°$

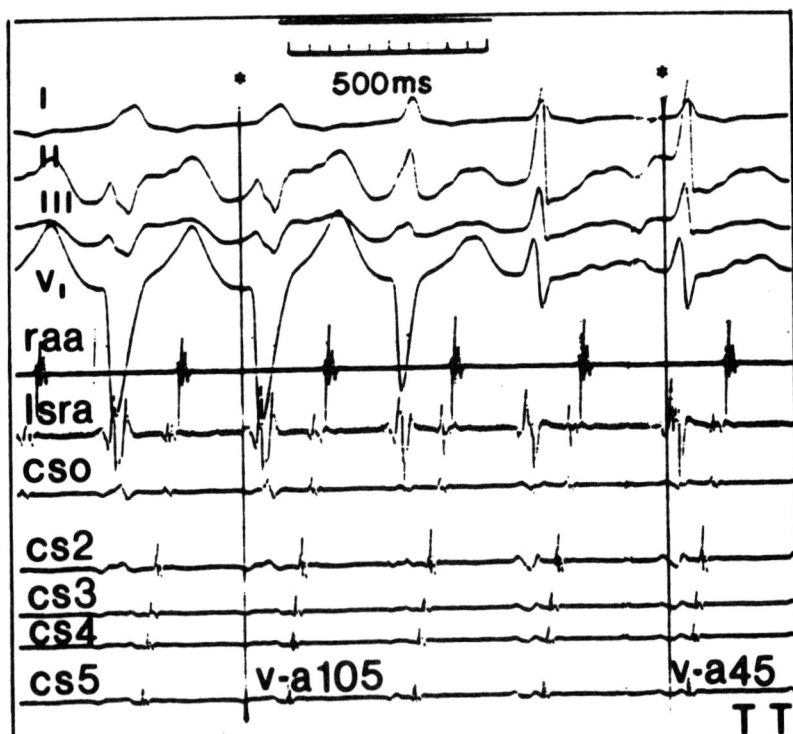

Figure 7C.

Comment:

Since this is the same patient as #5, identification of the tachycardia mechanism is clear from the last three beats of the ECG, that is orthodromic reciprocating tachycardia utilizing a left free wall accessory pathway. The first seven beats show left bundle-branch block with a longer tachycardia cycle length compared to the narrow QRS portion of the tachycardia. This provides a clue to the left free wall location of the retrograde limb of the circuit [Table I, step 9b]. In the presence of left bundle-branch block the retrograde ventriculoatrial interval is necessarily prolonged by the intervention of left bundle-branch block in patients with a left sided free wall accessory pathway. Therefore as left bundle-branch block disappears, the ventriculoatrial interval shortens and the tachycardia accelerates, cycle length shortening by about 30 msec.

The intracardiac recordings shown in Figure 7C confirm these findings. Following the first two QRS complexes showing left bundle-branch block with left axis deviation, the ventriculoatrial interval is 105 msec. After normalization of the QRS the ventriculoatrial interval shortens to 45 msec. Note the atrial activation sequence beginning in the coronary sinus 5 cm within the orifice, activating later the septum and right atrial appendage, and that the sequence does not change as the tachycardia accelerates [Table I, step 11b].

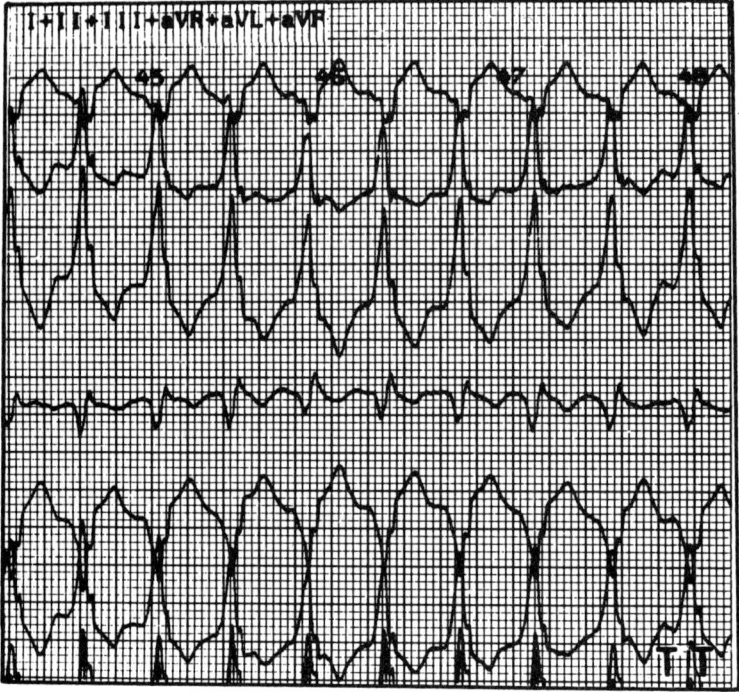

Figure 8A. 29-Year-Old Male.

Cycle length (msec): _____

Rate (bpm): _____

QRS duration (msec): _____

Regularity; Yes/No _____

  Group Beating? _____

P waves visible? Yes/No _____

P waves associated? Yes/No _____

  If so, long or short R-P? _____

  P wave vector: _____

Describe QRS morphology: V_1—V_6—

QRS axis: _____

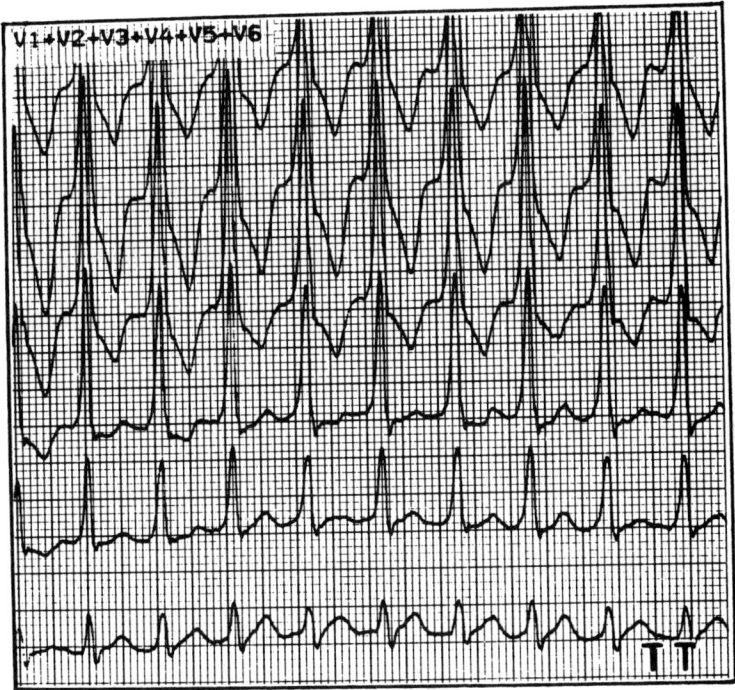

Figure 8B. No Heart Disease.

Probable arrhythmia diagnosis: _____
    If SVT, probable mechanism: _____
    If VT, probable site of origin: _____
Next diagnostic maneuver:
1. Vagal maneuver   [ ]
2. Atrial or esophageal electrogram   [ ]
3. Administration of verapamil, esmolol or
    adenosine   [ ]
4. Administration of lidocaine or procainamide   [ ]
5. Administration of atropine or isoproterenol   [ ]
6. Synchronized DC cardioversion   [ ]
7. His bundle recording   [ ]
8. Programmed stimulation   [ ]

Atrial Flutter with 2:1 Preexcited Response

Cycle length: 430 msec

Rate: 140 bpm

QRS: 160 msec

Regular

P waves visible. Atrial activity detectable. There is a positive deflection just before the QRS onset in lead I and there is a positive or biphasic deflection just after the QRS complex in leads II and III.

QRS morphology: Preexcited QRS with delta wave forces oriented rightward, anteriorly and inferiorly. R in V_1, Rs in V_6.

QRS axis: 110°

Comment:

The diagnosis of this tachycardia is extremely difficult from the surface ECG alone. Since this comes from the same patient as in the foregoing examples, the pattern of full preexcitation will now be familiar. Faced with this electrocardiogram at first presentation in an emergency room, the differential diagnosis would include the following: (1) ventricular tachycardia, (2) atrial tachycardia with 1 :1 preexcited response, (3) atrial flutter with 2 :1 preexcited response, (4) antidromic reciprocating tachycardia, utilizing a left free wall accessory pathway as the anterograde limb, and the atrioventricular node as the retrograde limb (5) reciprocating tachycardia utilizing two accessory pathways, the anterograde limb being a left free wall accessory pathway, (6) supraventricular tachycardia of a variety of mechanisms with atypical right bundle-branch block [Table I, step 9c].

The correct diagnosis rests on the identification of atrial activity. Although it is not completely certain from the surface electrocardiogram atrial activity can be suspected by noting the positive deflections preceding the QRS onset in lead I and the biphasic deflections just following the QRS complex in lead II. If these represent atrial activity, then the calculated atrial cycle length is approximately 215 msec, half the ventricular cycle length. This suggests atrial flutter with 2 :1 atrioventricular response via a left free wall accessory pathway. At the bedside it would be difficult to make this diagnosis without the aid of atrial electrograms [Table I, step 9d]. Vagal maneuvers are not likely to slow the ventricular response via the accessory pathway. Administration of lidocaine or procainamide may block the accessory pathway or prolong the accessory pathway refractory period allowing identification of the flutter activity in the baseline [Table II, step 4, 7]. Recording of an esophageal or atrial electrogram is the only certain way of making the correct diagnosis in this case. Intracardiac recordings shown in Figure 8C demonstrate atrial flutter with a slightly irregular atrial cycle length averaging 210 msec. The slightly irregular ventricular response averages 420 msec establishing the 2 :1 relationship [Table I, step 5b].

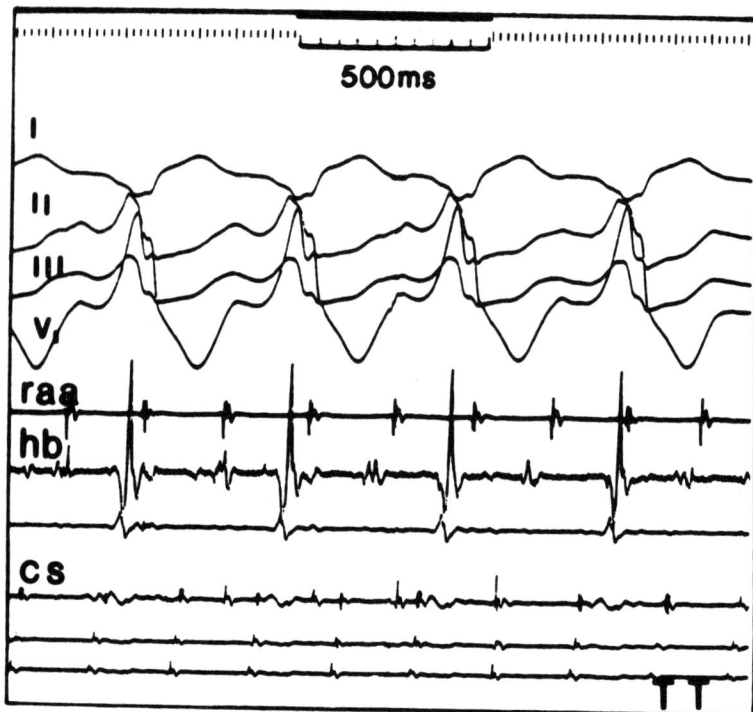

Figure 8C.

Figures 8D and 8E on pages 74 and 75 are from the same patient at another time.

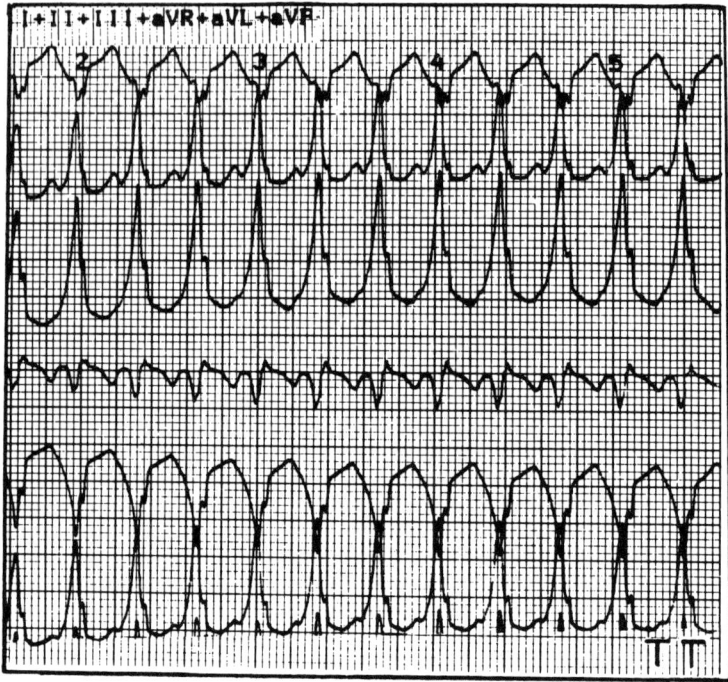

Figure 8D.

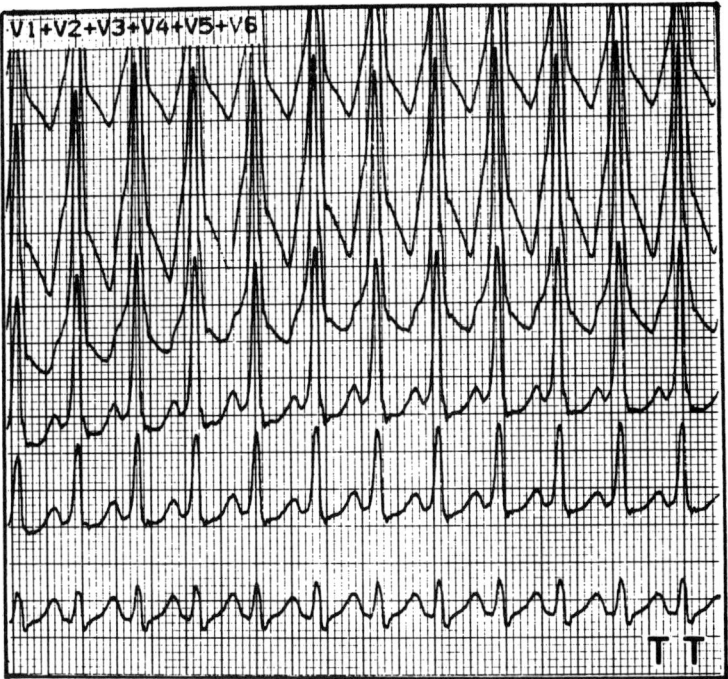

Figure 8E.

Comment:

In Figures 8D and 8E a similar tachycardia is shown. The cycle length is 345 msec. Atrial activity cannot be discerned reliably. Intracardiac recordings (not shown) confirmed the nature of this tachycardia to be antidromic reciprocating tachycardia in which the retrograde limb was the normal atrioventricular conduction system. The cycle length of 345 msec is too short to suggest atrial flutter with 2 :1 atrioventricular conduction, too long to be consistent with atrial flutter with 1 :1 conduction but would also be an appropriate cycle length for an intraatrial tachycardia with 1 :1 preexcited response [Table I, step 9c, 11d].

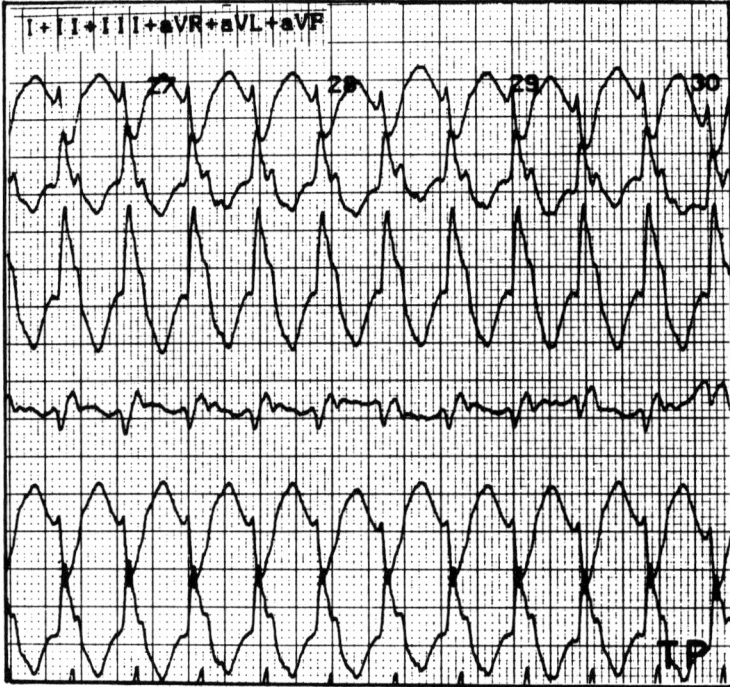

Figure 9A. 64-Year-Old Male.

Cycle length (msec):   _____
Rate (bpm):   _____
QRS duration (msec):   _____
Regularity; Yes/No   _____
    Group Beating?   _____
P waves visible? Yes/No   _____
P waves associated? Yes/No   _____
    If so, long or short R-P?   _____
    P wave vector: _____
Describe QRS morphology: V_1—V_6—
QRS axis: _____

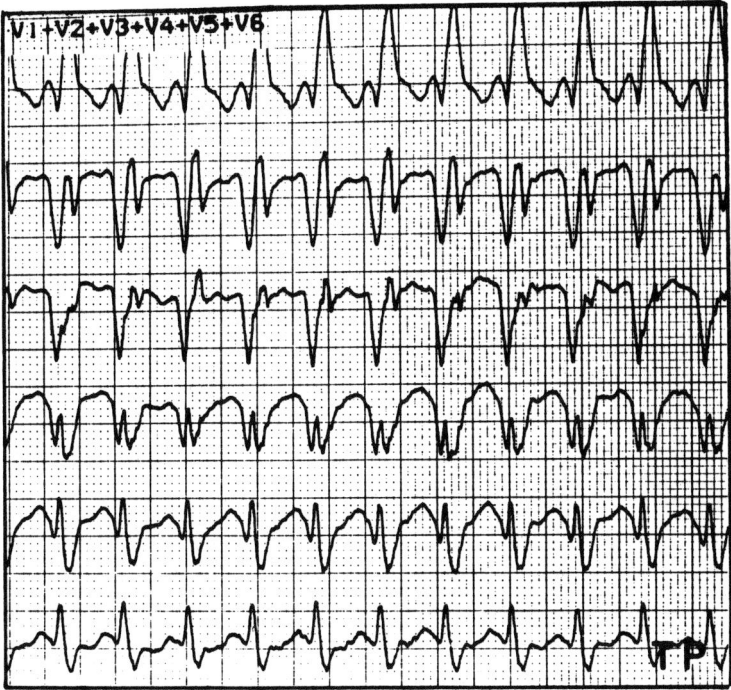

Figure 9B. Previous Myocardial Infarction.

Probable arrhythmia diagnosis: _____
   If SVT, probable mechanism: _____
   If VT, probable site of origin: _____
Next diagnostic maneuver:
1. Vagal maneuver   [ ]
2. Atrial or esophageal electrogram   [ ]
3. Administration of verapamil, esmolol or
    adenosine   [ ]
4. Administration of lidocaine or procainamide   [ ]
5. Administration of atropine or isoproterenol   [ ]
6. Synchronized DC cardioversion   [ ]
7. His bundle recording   [ ]
8. Programmed stimulation   [ ]

Sustained Ventricular Tachycardia
Cycle length: 440 msec
Rate: 136 bpm
QRS: 185 msec
Regular
P waves visible sporadically during the tachycardia, for example just after the QRS following the label 27 and just before the QRS labelled 30, indicating atrioventricular dissociation [Table I, step 5c].
QRS morphology: Generally resembles right bundle-branch block, in being inscribed anteriorly and rightward, but has broad initial Q waves in leads V_2 through V_6. The author prefers to describe the QRS as follows: rsR in V_1; qRS in V_6. Note that the biphasic deflections at the end of the QRS in V_3 and V_4 are not retrograde P waves but part of the QRS itself.
QRS axis: 120°

Comment:

In this case, comparison with the previous ECG in sinus rhythm was revealing (Figure 9C). This showed "anteroseptal" Q waves, V_1 through V_3 with bifascicular block (right bundle-branch block and left anterior fascicular block). The marked changes in frontal plane axis and the QRS conformation different from classical right bundle-branch block during the tachycardia both supported the diagnosis of ventricular tachycardia [Table I, step 10b]. It has been pointed out by others, that since ventricular tachycardia usually emanates from a site adjacent to a previous myocardial infarct, the initial QRS vector of the tachycardia frequently resembles that of the QRS during sinus rhythm, i.e., the ventricular tachycardia "remembers" the site of infarction. In this case, the initial QRS vector during tachycardia proceeds posteriorly, directly inferiorly and generally away from the apex (q in V_6) consistent with a site of initial ventricular activation in the anteroapical area of the left ventricle. This site was confirmed by intraoperative endocardial mapping.

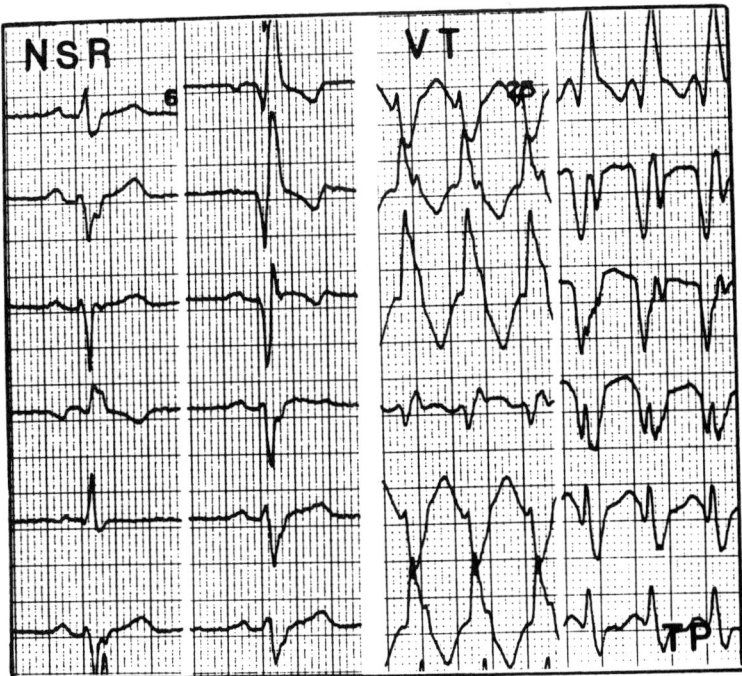

Figure 9C.

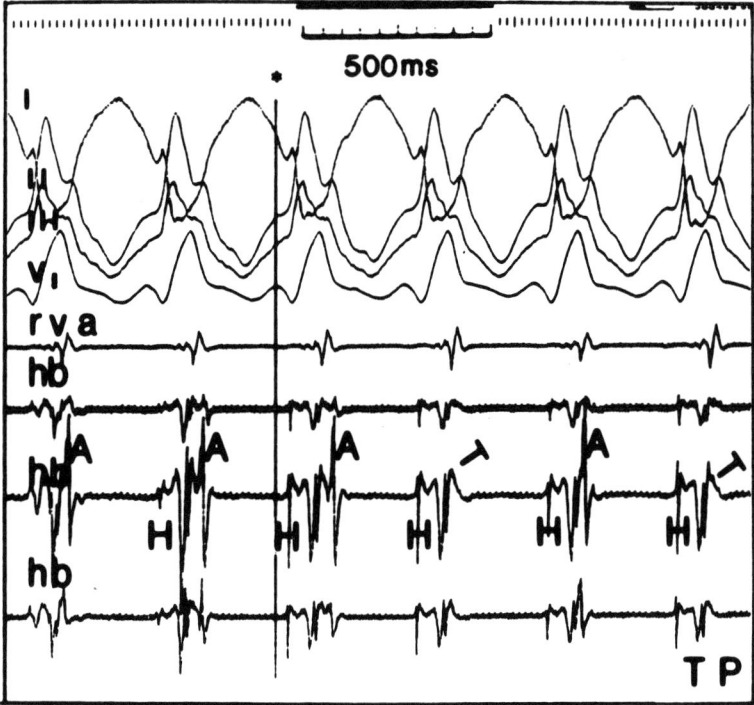

Figure 9D.

Intracardiac recordings (Figure 9D) taken at another time show type I retrograde second-degree ventriculoatrial block during ventricular tachycardia which was reproduced during programmed ventricular stimulation. The ventriculoatrial intervals increase by only small increments in the first three beats of the panel. Note, however, the measurable shortening of the ventriculoatrial interval following the fifth QRS (with similar atrial electrogram morphology) establishing the type of second-degree block as type I [Table I, step 5c]. The recording of His bundle deflections during ventricular tachycardia is not uncommon [Table I, step 11a]. In this example the V-H interval measured 35 msec. Since the activation during tachycardia began in the anteroapical left ventricle, retrograde propagation to the His bundle can be presumed to have occurred via the left anterior fascicle.

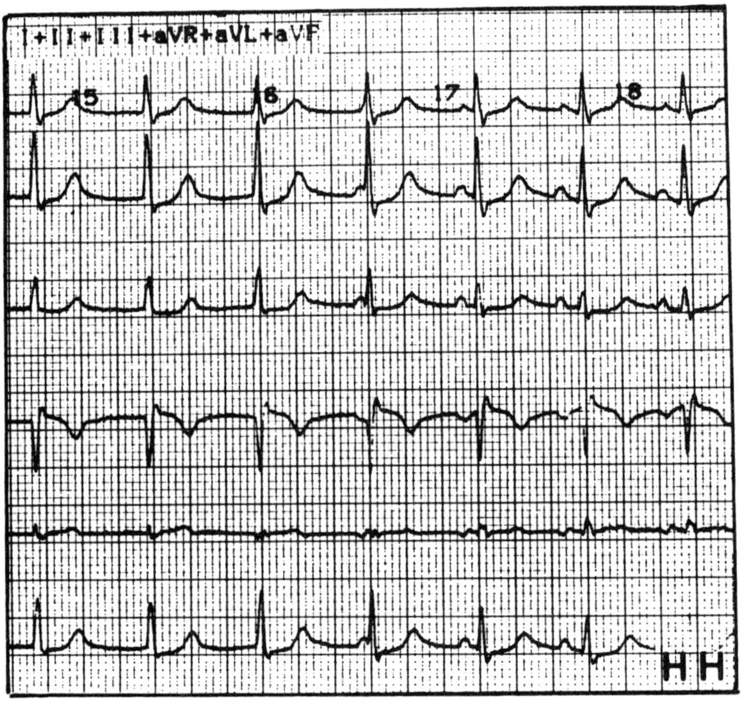

Figure 10A. 25-Year-Old Female.

Cycle length (msec): _____
Rate (bpm): _____
QRS duration (msec): _____
Regularity; Yes/No _____
  Group Beating? _____
P waves visible? Yes/No _____
P waves associated? Yes/No _____
  If so, long or short R-P? _____
  P wave vector: _____
Describe QRS morphology: V_1—V_6—
QRS axis: _____

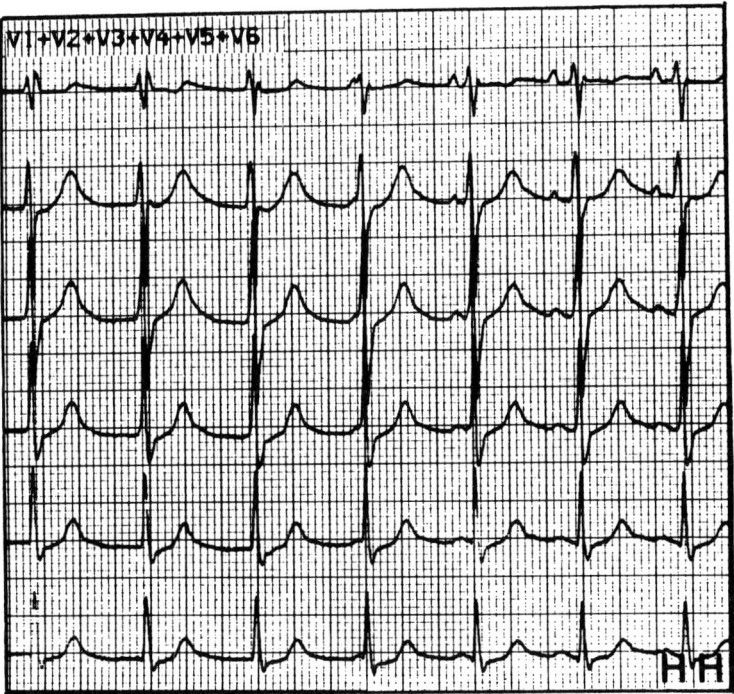

Figure 10B. No Heart Disease.

Probable arrhythmia diagnosis: _____
   If SVT, probable mechanism: _____
   If VT, probable site of origin: _____
Next diagnostic maneuver:
1. Vagal maneuver   [ ]
2. Atrial or esophageal electrogram   [ ]
3. Administration of verapamil, esmolol or
   adenosine   [ ]
4. Administration of lidocaine or procainamide   [ ]
5. Administration of atropine or isoproterenol   [ ]
6. Synchronized DC cardioversion   [ ]
7. His bundle recording   [ ]
8. Programmed stimulation   [ ]

Accelerated Junctional Rhythm with Isorhythmic Atrioventricular Dissociation
Cycle length: 640 to 560 msec
Rate: 94 to 107 bpm
QRS: 80 msec
Regular, until the last beat, which is early, representing capture of the ventricles by a sinus P wave. P waves are superimposed on the QRS appearing as a "pseudo-R-prime" in V_1 in the first three beats. Sinus P waves gradually accelerate and emerge in front of the QRS. Note that loss of the "pseudo-R-prime" in V_1 occurs in the last four beats.
QRS morphology: Normal in capture beats.
QRS axis: 60°

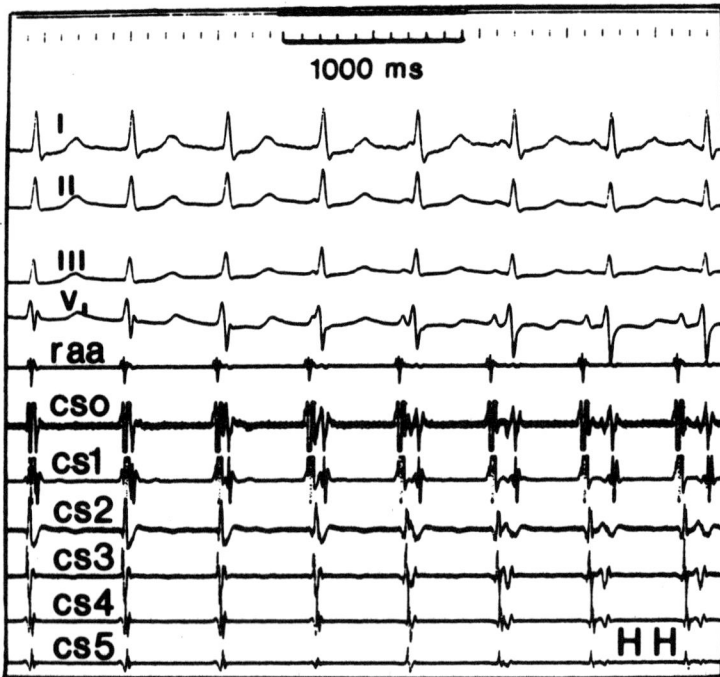

Figure 10C.

Comment:

The intracardiac recordings (Figure 10C) demonstrate the timing of P waves and their contribution to the summated forces during the QRS. If the atria had been captured retrogradely via the atrioventricular node during accelerated junctional rhythm the P wave vector would usually be oriented superiorly and anteriorly, manifested by a positive P in V_1 (present) and a negative P in lead III. During the last four beats when the P wave has advanced in front of the QRS, the QRS complexes show an S wave in lead III. The absence of the S wave in the first two beats suggests that the representation of the P wave in these beats must be a positive deflection cancelling the S wave. Thus, it can be presumed that the origin of P waves throughout the tracing is from the sinus node and that retrograde activation of the atria from the junctional focus is not present [Table I, step 4]. Thus isorhythmic atrioventricular dissociation can be presumed. In cases of accelerated junctional rhythm where isorhythmic atrioventricular dissociation is not present (ie, 1 :1 retrograde atrial capture is present), it is useful to attempt to bring about a change in atrial or junctional rate by bedside maneuvers such as carotid sinus massage or isometric exercise which may dissociate the atria from the junction and permit a diagnosis to be made [Table II, step 4, 5]. This patient was taking oral verapamil, probably accounting for the lack of retrograde conduction. Accelerated junctional rhythm has been reported to be due to verapamil.

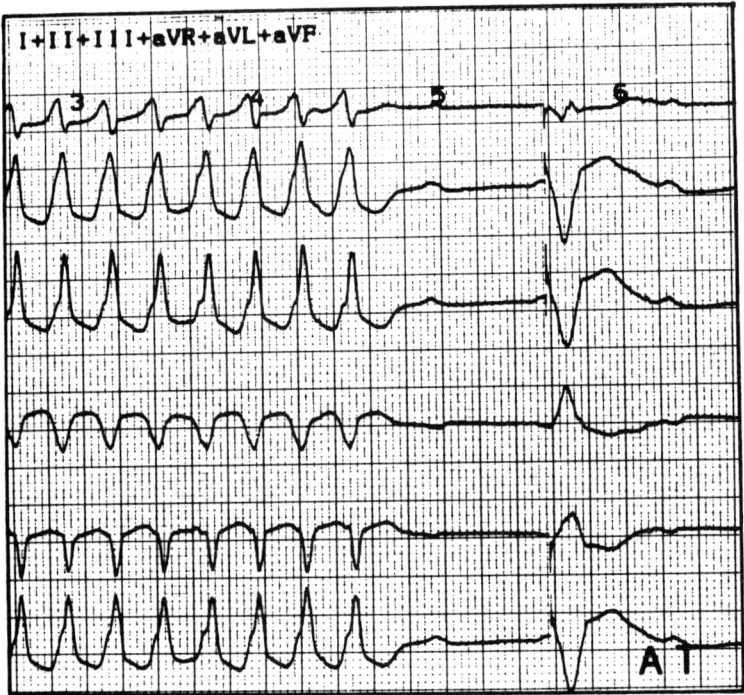

Figure 11A. 52-Year-Old Male.

Cycle length (msec):   _____
Rate (bpm):   _____
QRS duration (msec):   _____
Regularity; Yes/No   _____
    Group Beating?   _____
P waves visible? Yes/No   _____
P waves associated? Yes/No   _____
    If so, long or short R-P?   _____
    P wave vector: _____
Describe QRS morphology: V_1—V_6—
QRS axis: _____

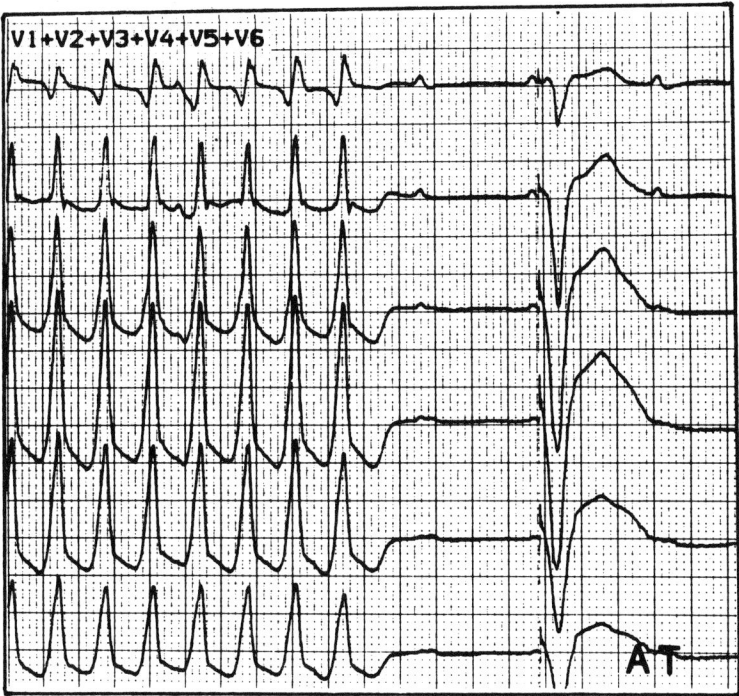

Figure 11B. Idiopathic Congestive Cardiomyopathy.

Probable arrhythmia diagnosis: _____
   If SVT, probable mechanism: _____
   If VT, probable site of origin: _____
Next diagnostic maneuver:
1. Vagal maneuver   [ ]
2. Atrial or esophageal electrogram   [ ]
3. Administration of verapamil, esmolol or
   adenosine   [ ]
4. Administration of lidocaine or procainamide   [ ]
5. Administration of atropine or isoproterenol   [ ]
6. Synchronized DC cardioversion   [ ]
7. His bundle recording   [ ]
8. Programmed stimulation   [ ]

Paroxysmal Ventricular Tachycardia with Atrioventricular Block

Cycle length: 265 msec
Rate: 226 bpm
QRS: 140 msec
Regular
P waves visible, dissociated. P wave vector downward, leftward and anteriorly [Table I, step 4, 5].
QRS morphology: QR in V_1, R in V_6.
QRS axis: 80°

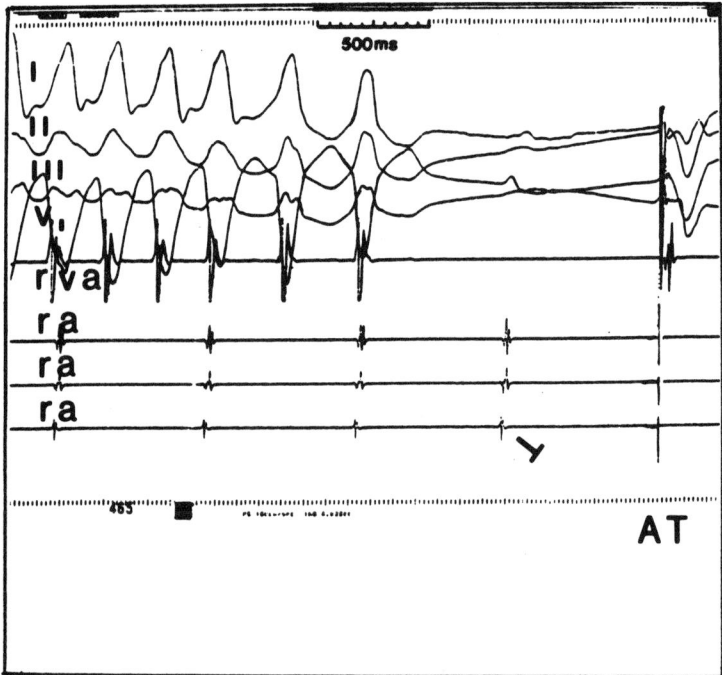

Figure 11C.

Comment:

The main point to take from this example is that the presence of atrioventricular block as seen after termination of this tachycardia, virtually excludes any possibility of the tachycardia being supraventricular in mechanism. This is simply a function of the fact that all forms of supraventricular tachycardia utilize all or part of the atrioventricular conduction system as an essential part of the mechanism of the tachycardia. For all practical purposes, the only form of supraventricular tachycardia that could exist in the same patient who has atrioventricular block during sinus rhythm would be junctional ectopic focus tachycardia in a patient with atrioventricular nodal block.

That this tachycardia is ventricular is also confirmed by the QRS duration of 140 msec [Table I, step 1], and the presence of atrioventricular dissociation, best seen in leads aVL and $V_1 - V_4$. This example also makes the point that if a single lead had been used to make a diagnosis in this tachycardia, one could have been seriously misled about the QRS duration; for example lead aVL looks narrow on casual inspection. Simultaneous recording of multiple ECG leads leaves no doubt that the QRS is wide. In the precordial leads the QR pattern in V_1 is highly suggestive of ventricular tachycardia [Table I, step 10b].

The intracardiac recordings of the last few cycles of an episode of induced ventricular tachycardia are shown (Figure 11C). These recordings demonstrate the presence of atrioventricular dissociation during the tachycardia and atrioventricular block during subsequent sinus rhythm. This patient's tachycardia was resistant to standard antiarrhythmic drugs and he was placed on amiodarone which successfully prevented tachycardia during follow up. The single-chambered demand pacemaker was revised to a dual-chambered system with substantial benefit to the patient in terms of effort tolerance.